What's Eating Your Child?

The Hidden Connections Between Food and Childhood Ailments: Anxiety, Recurrent Ear Infections, Stomachaches, Picky Eating, Rashes, ADHD, and More. **And What Every Parent Can Do About It.**

Kelly Dorfman, MS, LND

WORKMAN PUBLISHING ▪ NEW YORK

To Jeff, Ben, Isabel, Tory, and Tania

Library of Congress Cataloging-in-Publication Data is available.

ISBN 978-0-7611-6119-6

Cover typography by Chris Tobias
Design by Sara Edward-Corbett
Author photo by Lee Love

Workman books are available at special discount when purchased in bulk for premiums and sales promotions as well as for fund-raising or educational use. Special editions or book excerpts can also be created to specification. For details, contact the Special Sales Director at the address below, or send an e-mail to specialmarkets@workman.com.

Workman Publishing Company, Inc.
225 Varick Street
New York, NY 10014-4381
www.workman.com

Printed in the United States of America

First Printing March 2011

10 9 8 7 6 5 4 3 2 1

ABOUT THE STORIES IN THIS BOOK

All of the cases, stories, and people in this book are real. The names of the children and parents have been changed and some identifying details altered to protect the privacy of those with whom I have had the privilege to work. In addition, some of the stories represent a piece of a more complicated situation.

The conversations with clients were reconstructed from my notes and memory. I attempted to accurately reflect the tenor and content of the interchanges, but the wording is not exact. The quotes from doctors, professionals, and research, however, are precise.

I wish to thank all of my clients and families whose stories I am sharing. May they enrich your life as much as they have enriched mine.

★ ★ ★

ABOUT THE ADVICE IN THIS BOOK

This book contains the opinions and ideas of its author and is not meant in either its parts or its entirety to be a substitute for medical advice. It is intended to provide helpful information on the subjects addressed in its pages and is offered with the understanding that the author and publisher are not engaged in rendering medical, health, or any other kind of personal professional services. The reader should consult a competent medical professional before applying or adopting any of the suggestions in this book or drawing any inferences from them. The author and publisher disclaim all responsibility for any liability or risk that is incurred as a consequence, directly or indirectly, from the use or application of any of the contents of this book.

Acknowledgments

I WOULD LIKE TO THANK THE following wonderful people:

Peter Steinberg, the best book agent on the planet, who asked me to write a book and then helped me do it. Much of this help came in the form of Billie Fitzpatrick, my collaborator. She was full of enthusiasm and helpful advice for the project from beginning to end and is a wizard with words.

A large group of brilliant and supportive physicians and researchers, including Dr. Marilyn Agin, Dr. Michael Firestone, Dr. Mark Freilich, the late Dr. Stanley Greenspan, Dr. Richard Layton, Dr. John Merendino Jr., Dr. Claudia Morris, Dr. Charlie Olsen, Dr. Maurine Packard, Dr. Celia Padron, Dr. Neil Spiegel, Dr. Ioana Razi, and Dr. Anju Usman. If all doctors were like these people, we would not be having a health care crisis.

An even larger group of gifted and clever clinicians with whom I have had the astounding pleasure to work with, play with, and borrow ideas from: Dr. Lynn Balzer Martin, Lindsey Biel, Dr. Dee Blanco, Christy Kennedy Bosarge, Dr. Barbara Dunbar, Dr. Catherine Fitzgerald, Dr. Jane Koomar, Valerie DeJean, Lynn Grodzki, Dana Laake, Maude

La Roux, Dianne Lazer, Patty Lemer, Deb Motley, Dr. Kathy Platzman, Suzanne Scurlock, Paula Stewart, Shelley Stravitz, June Sussman, Bobbe Wade, Victoria Wood, and Lauren Zimet. If these women do not rule the world, they should.

My sage and trusty network of friends and family who have been invaluable with their support, ideas, and encouragement: Hannah Quinn Bleicher, Susan Beram, Tania Celii, Leni Gurin, Sally Klinkon, Catherine Lisson, Beverley Martin, Loretta McMahon, Frances Pollak, and Joan Wofford.

Margot Herrera, my editor; Beth Wareham, the director of publicity; Rebecca Carlisle, publicist; and the other creative forces and all-around pleasant people at Workman Publishing.

The clients whose stories I have used but whose names will have to remain a closely guarded secret. One exception of someone not in the book is David Katz, who has sent me reams of useful data, books, and articles through the years, some of which came in mighty handy.

Last but certainly not least are my husband, Jeff, and children, Ben, Isabel, and Tory. They have been willing, if not always enthusiastic, guinea pigs through the years for countless new nutrition experiments. Every supplement and diet change in this book has been tried by at least one of them. They have also helped me in various important ways during this process, everything from setting up radio interviews to operating as my own personal computer geek. I could not have done this, and probably would not have wanted to, without all of you.

Contents

The Art of Medicine

BY DR. RICHARD E. LAYTON,
PEDIATRIC ALLERGY SPECIALIST

R EADING THIS BOOK CAUSED ME to reflect on my career in medicine. Looking back to medical school and my residency, I felt I was very well-trained in the science of medicine. I received an excellent education in diagnosing diseases based on an abnormal lab test, X-ray, or biopsy, and learned how to treat them with medication. I was taught to recognize the symptoms of many illnesses, to know when someone needed surgery, and how to tell if a situation was an emergency. These were the priorities. The result: Doctors, such as myself, are better at treating disease than looking for its underlying cause. In other words, we're well trained in the science—but not the art—of medicine.

In my opinion, when a medical problem is subjective and there are no lab tests to confirm a diagnosis, many patients receive substandard care.

For example, if a patient complains of multiple gastrointestinal symptoms, which could include bloating, erratic bowel movements, and heartburn, but his gastrointestinal workup, including endoscopy, colonoscopy, and various sonograms, yields normal results, he is often told, "You have irritable bowel syndrome." Essentially, the doctor is saying,

"I have not found the specific cause of your problems, so this is your diagnosis."

The same holds true for a patient who complains of fatigue: If her lab work comes back negative, she is told, "You have chronic fatigue syndrome." Similarly, a patient who has muscle and joint pain but does not test positive for an autoimmune disorder such as lupus is told, "You have fibromyalgia."

There really are patients with irritable bowel syndrome, chronic fatigue syndrome, and fibromyalgia, but it's my belief that at least 80 percent of patients who receive these diagnoses actually have undiagnosed complaints that do not fit the science/disease model we learn in medical school.

I practiced primary care pediatrics from 1972 to 1987 before specializing in kids with allergies. When I found parents asking me, "Why is my child on so many antibiotics?" or "Does my child really need to be on Ritalin for ADHD?" I reassessed my medical responsibilities. I started reading about underlying causes for medical problems (rather than focusing solely on the "solutions") and the more I read, the more I was concerned about the way I was practicing.

Two children changed my career: The first was a boy who complained of severe migraine headaches. I referred him appropriately to a very good pediatric neurologist who ran all the right tests and said that this child had "psychosomatic migraine headaches." By then, I had read that a craved food can be a problem food. I asked the boy's mother, "Is there any food your son eats every day?" She said, "He loves peanut butter." I said, "OK, take him off peanut butter (and all peanut products) for ten days and give me a call back." When I received the call, I was delighted to find out that the boy had not had a migraine the entire ten days, compared to daily migraines while ingesting peanut butter daily.

The second patient was a girl with severe abdominal pain. After running a number of tests and still not having a sense of what the problem could be, I actually admitted her into the hospital at the convenience of not only myself but also the gastroenterologist, psychiatrist, and other

"-ologists." Nobody came up with an answer except for psychosomatic abdominal pain. After the hospitalization, I read that milk can be a problem food. When I asked the girl's mother, "How much milk does your daughter drink?" she said, "Oh, she drinks four glasses a day." I said, "Take her off all milk for ten days and give me a call." Surprise—no abdominal pain for those ten days.

We need to get away from the one-size-fits-all "it's a virus" response to hard-to-categorize illnesses. Even though that may be the correct diagnosis most of the time, it should not be an assumption. Likewise, when a parent raises concerns about her son's development at eighteen months, we doctors need to refrain from automatically saying, "You are stressed out, let's wait," or "He's a boy—they develop later," or "He's a second child," and assuming that that is the answer. Even if the doctor is right ninety-nine times out of a hundred, Kelly and I are seeing the one-hundredth child.

Over the past fifteen years that I have been working with Kelly, I have been amazed at how intuitive and bright she is. She is a true Sherlock Holmes. Her ability to listen to a history and use her common sense, brain, and intuition to determine the source of a problem is truly remarkable. She has taught me an enormous amount about nutrition and how important the right diet and supplements are to attain optimal health. When it comes to the patients in my practice, I have more confidence in Kelly's opinion than that of anyone else in medicine. She is brilliant.

This book is "must-reading" for parents and doctors. If our medical model incorporated its premises, there is no doubt in my mind that we would waste less money on lab tests and medications that don't solve children's health problems, and at the same time we would raise healthier, happier kids.

Introduction

HAVE YOU EVER WONDERED WHY your son keeps getting ear infections? Are you uncomfortable giving him so many antibiotics? Does your child look pale and pasty and get sick often? Have you ever worried that your moody daughter who lives on pasta and apple juice is malnourished, despite your doctor's assurance that she's fine because she's "on the growth chart"? Have you ever suspected that your son's inattentiveness may have something to do with how little he sleeps and how much sugary food he eats? These concerns may seem difficult to address and like part of everyday parenthood, but they can disrupt the fabric of a child's (and a family's) life.

For the past twenty-nine years, I've been working directly with the families of thousands of children of all ages—from newborn babies to teenagers to kids home from college—fielding such questions about the reasons behind seemingly innocuous but otherwise "untreatable" childhood behaviors and conditions. These children are referred to me by their stymied physicians, frustrated specialists, concerned teachers, and other parents of children with whom I've worked, as well as by word of mouth that seems to have spread from the East Coast to the West. The average family in my practice has consulted between three and five medical experts before seeking my advice. They come to me because they have reached the end of the line with ineffective treatments for their child's ailments and need a new, more successful way to approach his or her health problems. Indeed, the bodies of today's children are under fire from environmental pollutants, additives in processed food, viruses messing up their developing neurological systems, and reactions to commonplace foods that can cause behavioral, psychological, and physical symptoms. This generation of children has the highest rate of food allergies, obesity, behavioral and emotional disorders, autoimmune disease, and learning issues ever recorded.

What have I been offering to these children and their concerned parents? Simple yet scientifically supported nutritional solutions that address, mitigate, and sometimes even erase both the symptoms and the causes of such stubborn health problems as food allergies, reflux, constipation, picky eating, attention issues, moodiness, behavioral difficulties, lack of energy, sleeplessness, and learning disabilities.

Of course, you will not be surprised to know that as a nutritionist with decades of experience, I believe in the power of good foods, vitamins, and minerals to create better health, growth, and development in children. But what may be unfamiliar to you is the degree to which nutrition plays a role in healing ordinary conditions and extraordinary situations—from earwax buildup to reflux, from temper tantrums to chronic tummy aches, from odd social behavior to pervasive anxiety. Yes, in many cases these situations stem from nutritional deficiencies or negative reactions to certain food groups.

Many years ago when I first began realizing the extent of the nutrition crisis in our country's children, I was distraught. Why weren't families getting proper nutrition advice? Was our health care system so backward that it couldn't provide essential, scientifically supported nutrition information to parents? I took this frustration and decided to channel it for good: I not only began to delve into the most cutting-edge, published research on the effect of nutrition on behavioral, emotional, physical, and learning issues that commonly occur in children, but I cofounded a nonprofit organization called Developmental Delay Resources to help parents and professionals find safe biological treatments for attention, behavioral, and cognitive issues. I was committed to taking on this challenge and reaching as many of these kids as possible. And even though many of the children I've treated have experienced remarkable recoveries, I know there are thousands more out there who need this same information. It's for this reason that I have written this book.

> *What's Eating Your Child?* is for parents who want to be proactive participants in their children's health, confident about and able to implement the most cutting-edge, scientifically supported nutritional advice available today.

What's Eating Your Child? is for those of you who have been looking for a way to navigate and sort through all the new information about nutrition—from omega-3 fatty acids to vitamin C. As parents, we are inundated with nutritional information, but no single place succinctly applies it to specific childhood health concerns.

What do I do exactly? I teach parents how to think about health and become the chief investigator in the unsolved mystery behind their child's elusive condition. In most cases, these children not only experience a reversal of debilitating symptoms but discover the power they have over their own health—all by adding missing vitamins or minerals, avoiding foods that their bodies can't tolerate, or taking a supplement that their brains need to function properly.

What's Eating Your Child? is for parents who want to be proactive participants in their children's health, confident about and able to implement the most cutting-edge, scientifically supported nutritional advice available today. It's also for those of you who want alternatives to relying on over-the-counter medicines and prescriptions that may or may not work and have their own side effects. If you feel in your gut that something is upsetting your child's stomach or affecting his ability to sleep, calm down, or focus, then you are probably right. And the strategies and insights that I've gathered here will enable you to follow that gut feeling and find real, healthy ways to get your child on the right track so he can grow—physically, emotionally, and intellectually—to his full potential. This nutritional advice can truly change your child's health destiny!

A FEW THINGS TO KNOW ABOUT THIS BOOK

W*hat's Eating your Child?* is very practical; it shows you how to uncover the clues behind your child's health problem and find an accurate, nutritional treatment—immediately. This book does not take on every single disease or ailment that can occur to your child; rather it focuses on those that can be treated (or reversed) with nutrition. You will find stories from my case files that will help you follow the clues to unravel symptoms such as the following:

- chronic ear infections
- rough, patchy skin and eczema
- picky eating
- earwax buildup
- chronic stomachaches, constipation, and diarrhea
- lack of growth and delayed development
- attention problems, including both dreaminess and hyperactivity
- speech delays
- weird social behavior
- temper tantrums, mood swings, and other mood and behavioral problems

Each case also highlights a core principle that you as parents can use as a general guideline when beginning to understand and then address your child's situation. These principles will empower and guide you as you become more comfortable with the process of detecting, identifying, and then finding the best way to address your child's health problem.

Even though you can certainly jump to a specific chapter that relates to a current condition that is affecting your child, I encourage you to read the book cover to cover. You will find all sorts of information that you never realized could help cure the constant tummy aches your ten-year-old complains about or finally settle down your hyper eight-year-old before he drives you all crazy. Like a crime scene investigation show, these stories from my case files are entertaining, but they can also empower you to take control of your child's health in a profound new way. Unlike TV crime dramas, the perpetrator here is usually edible or the crime is one of omission. Best of all, the stories are all true.

I always keep in mind that sometimes there's a nutritional solution to the problem and sometimes there isn't. When people ask me how I know what works, I always respond, "Trial and terror." It takes an adventuresome spirit to take the road less traveled and address your child's diet—especially if she is already giving you a hard time about eating in general. (For that picky eater, you will find my E.A.T. program—a time-tested, completely practical way to help your child open her mind to new foods and slowly but surely integrate more healthy choices into her diet.)

As I mentioned at the outset, many of the parents with whom I work begin this process with a bit of trepidation. Although the ideas are exciting and potentially life-changing, doubts may begin to surface. "What if my doctor objects?" "I worry that I will be experimenting on my own children." Or as one mother nervously asked me recently, "How can I get the grandparents on board? They'll never understand how dairy can be bad and will never support taking it out of their grandchild's diet." Indeed, I know from experience that when a parent says, "I don't want to experiment on my child" that is code for "I'm not comfortable with this idea yet." Luckily, it is hard to do serious damage by either removing certain foods from a diet or by adding nutritional supplements but relatively easy to reassure parents with scientific evidence and thoughtful consideration of their concerns.

Rest assured that you will find real-life ways to implement these changes with your kids at home, and I will offer you specific instructions on which steps to take first and how to speak with your doctor or health care provider, as well as other considerations as you begin this process. Within each case and throughout each chapter, you will also find strategies and insights to help you manage the doubters, naysayers, and resisters in your life, including yourself.

KNOW YOURSELF

L et's start with you. Raising a child is one big uncontrolled experiment, and as parents we can experience any change to our routine as bothersome, if not terrifying. A parent may not blink over a spinal tap in the ER but feel agitated and anxious about adding a vitamin supplement. Why? Because this parent does not yet have enough information to trust and have confidence in the power and safety of nutritional healing. But once you believe in your course of action, it's much easier to navigate the changes you are asking your child to make, especially when conflict ensues.

"Peter gets upset if I ask him to eat vegetables," a parent complains. Another admits, "I really don't like vegetables myself. How am I supposed to persuade Claire to eat them?" Throughout the book, you will find helpful strategies to get you over these bumps in the road. For instance, you can learn how to steel yourself in the face of an angry or hysterical outburst from your five-year-old who is resisting taking his vitamins. You can also learn to expand your own food repertoire to include one or two vegetables—perhaps this even becomes part of your daughter's process, something you do together. One bite a day for three weeks will get you to a new place with that food. I've seen these strategies work again and again, and they can work for you.

My colleagues sometimes say I'm more of a psychotherapist than a nutritionist because I spend so much of my time with families coaching them to try to implement these nutritional changes and strategies. The truth is, finding the right answer to your child's health problem is often straightforward. But making the change can be stressful and, in fact, the ultimate challenge. What's more, in certain cases, I am not afraid to call upon a small army of therapists, psychotherapists, support groups, and other parents to help struggling parents. In one situation, I was working with four sets of parents who had adopted children from drug-addicted mothers. These kids had unique challenges not usually discussed at the monthly PTA meeting. I conscripted the mom with the most experience to lead an informal support group. Each member benefited from hearing about the others' issues and learned from their attempts to improve their children's lives.

> Why not ask Grandma to help with a trial period of no dairy so she can also provide feedback?

I can say this from all my years of working with nutrition and families: Once parents get a taste of success (their child stops complaining about his near-constant stomachache, or he starts going to the bathroom regularly without the help of laxatives, or his mood suddenly but consistently transforms from Yosemite Sam to Care Bear), they will feel newly confident that they are doing what's best for their child. Of course, parents may still encounter the occasional doubting spouse or relative. When I can, I invite parents to arrange appointments for the uncertain party so he or she has the opportunity to voice concerns and ask questions. In the grandparent case mentioned earlier, the mother intuitively suspected that her son's frequent ear infections and illnesses were caused by dairy sensitivity, and her seven-month-old was already starting down the same road with a two-month-long antibiotics-resistant infection. Why not ask Grandma to help with a trial period of no dairy so she can also provide feedback? Does she think Jack is feeling or looking better? Involving doubters in the process is often a helpful (and savvy) way to gain their support.

You will discover quickly in the pages ahead that you are not alone in your worry and concern about seemingly common childhood problems. Together, we will not only find the best way to address your child's symptoms but also arm you with the courage, compassion, and confidence to lead your child—and your family—on a path of greater health and well-being.

Nutrition Detection at Work

CHAPTER 1

How Important Is Nutrition, Really?

F EW PARENTS START OUT WITH THE GOAL of feeding their children toaster pastries for breakfast and peanut butter crackers for lunch, yet an astonishing number (if my practice is any indication) end up there. How many exactly? Hard to say, because so many of them are hiding in shame. These are not uneducated people. They are doctors, lawyers, and professionals. One high-powered executive with a master's degree in business came to speak to me about her son whose diet consisted almost entirely of candy bars and pretzels. He was, no surprise, not functioning in school or at home, and the many medications they had tried were not working. She felt so guilty and was so defensive that I could not find a neutral area where we could have a conversation about how to help him. She heard every suggestion, no matter how mild, as a referendum on her mothering skills. "He won't do it!" she insisted. "I have tried."

The scenario of a typical diet gone bad starts at age two when a sleep-starved mother hands her red-faced, screaming toddler a cracker or cookie so he will just shut up. The action is not seen as a long-term solution but a rare treat for a bad day. But little crackers and cookies work like a charm for toddlers. They melt in the mouth, can be held in the hand (for maximum control)–they are like toddler crack. The baby is happy! He stopped fussing at church. At Grandma's birthday party everyone remarked on how well behaved he was.

Yes, he refused to eat lunch, but that was a special occasion, and aren't all toddlers picky? *No, they are not.* If you give them only the good food you want them to eat, they will eat good food. However, once salty or sweet food is introduced and the child is at an age when it's developmentally appropriate to assume some control over what he puts in his mouth, then a bad habit will unwittingly begin, and things will go downhill from there. If the snack food is in the house, the child quickly learns that he can refuse dinner and scream until the preferred food appears. Few of us have the energy or patience at six-thirty at night to deal with a hysterical child. Besides, the rest of the family is trying to eat dinner, and isn't it better for the baby to eat something–even if it is junky–than nothing? A good mother does not let her child go hungry, right?

The final mental argument is that fighting about food causes eating disorders. Isn't this back-and-forth arguing about what to eat harmful to a child? This is how good moms and dads, under the guise of not letting their child go hungry and avoiding food fights, lay the foundation for bad eating. The two-year-old, under the chemical influence of highly flavored food and heady with newfound personal power, self-selects his own diet from this time forward.

Radical solution: Don't have anything in the house you do not want your child to eat.

NUTRITION TO THE RESCUE

If there is one idea I want you to take away from this book, it's this: Nutrition is important. Not only does it help your child's brain and body develop to his optimal potential, but it enables your child to live a healthy life, maximizing energy and minimizing illness. Perhaps you accept as a fact that all kids get sick. Perhaps you've been led to believe that conditions such as reflux, ear infections, stomachaches, moodiness, difficulty controlling behavior, and learning problems are all "normal"—and in no way impair how children grow and learn.

You are about to discover that many of these so-called common childhood ailments are indeed avoidable or can be dealt with nutritionally before they disrupt proper development or lead to more complex medical problems. Now you may be wondering, "Is this one of those books that recommends mustard packs for stomachaches or makes you feel bad for not raising your own chickens?" Absolutely not. It is a book that will take you on an important journey. I will show you how to take the concept we all know, "You are what you eat," and use it to make simple dietary adjustments that can make your child happier, healthier, and generally easier to live with. Furthermore, this trip will be entertaining and interesting.

For the scientifically oriented, there will be supportive studies and data to prove I am not making this all up. What surprises me most after more than twenty-five years as a practicing nutrition detective is not the lack of information (though more is always needed) but the limited way nutrition science is turned into usable information. I am committed to changing that deficiency.

WHERE I COME FROM

I always like to know where an author I'm reading or specialist I'm working with is coming from. A good detective understands her own prejudices as well as those of her resources. I was born on a mayonnaise farm. Just kidding. That is an old joke in my family. You would have to go back a few generations to hit a farmer in my family, but you would not have to travel far to see the Pennsylvania Dutch influence. Both my mother and father could speak the language of the Amish, and my grandparents spoke it around us when they did not want us to know something. My fondest memories of my grandmother are of her digging up dandelions for dandelion salad (with bacon grease dressing) or frying doughnuts for Fastnacht Day. (Fastnacht Day is the day before Lent and in the Pennsylvania Dutch tradition is an excuse to make potato doughnuts. There was no religious component.)

My parents did not have a speck of old country in them, particularly my mother, who would sooner have gallbladder surgery than fry a doughnut. In fact, my mother wanted as little to do with food as possible. Her favorite cookbook was Peggy Bracken's *I Hate to Cook Book* (which was just reissued for its fiftieth anniversary). She frequently lamented that cooking and eating were a big waste of time. Her goal was to spend as little time as possible thinking about and preparing food, and she succeeded spectacularly. Our regular diet was pretty much made up of dried-out meat, potaotes, and canned vegetables. Like my mother, I hadn't given food very much thought. I just assumed that everybody ate potatoes five nights a week.

But there was an irony in my mother's lackluster relationship to food and cooking: She was more confident about nutrition than most parents are today. Fruit was good (and easy), but soda was only for special occasions. McDonald's (the only fast-food establishment around when I was young) was always to be avoided. Packaged cookies were not good for you, but eating ice cream every day was okay. (Ice cream was a major food group at our house and one of the few premade foods condoned because it was from cows and therefore nutritious.)

As soon as I turned sixteen and could drive, my household chore became doing the food shopping. Still, I did not become interested in nutrition until I went to college. I was home visiting and doing the food shopping (naturally) when I stumbled upon a book called *Sugar Blues* by William Duffy. It was a book written in the 1970s about how sugar was as addicting as cocaine and almost as bad for you. He advocated giving up refined sugar as a way to improve overall health.

This was a revolutionary idea, and I was at just the right time and age to grab on to it with vigor. Out went the sugar from my diet, and although I was always slender, I lost five pounds and my skin cleared up.

I looked and felt better than I ever had. Within a short period of time, I had shifted majors and changed universities and was on my way to changing people's lives with nutrition.

Unfortunately, neither college nor grad school taught me how to apply nutritional science to people's lives; in fact, it became immediately clear that there was a primary disconnect in the field of clinical nutrition. Although there is endless talk about how important nutrition is, in practice, most of my professors rarely acted like it was that significant. Sure, if a person is obese or severely underweight or diabetic, a dietitian is called in. Otherwise, nutrition, although always stressed as important, is given only cursory consideration in the medical field. Those of us who believed more could be done with nutrition ended up working at health food stores or were labeled extremists.

> Although there is endless talk about how important nutrition is, in practice, most of my professors rarely acted like it was that significant.

Every field has its quirks, and in nutrition it is this lack of practical application of what we know about nutritional science. For example, any basic nutrition text will tell you that a primary symptom of zinc deficiency is poor growth. Yet in twenty-five years, I have never seen a regular pediatrician or endocrinologist test the blood-zinc levels of a child whose diagnosis is failure to thrive. Hormone levels and bone age will be evaluated but not zinc. The doctors are usually well trained and know zinc is necessary for growth hormone production. In many cases the parent will be distressed about the child's poor diet (a further hint that nutrition may be a factor), and still the test has not been run.

This does not make sense to me. One basic law of physics says that you cannot make matter from nothing. You have to start with something. In the case of the body, its ability to create must start from what it takes in or is born with. In other words, any growing, healing, development, and functioning you accomplish must evolve from what you come with, eat, drink, or breathe. You are born with about seven pounds of matter that will expand into a hundred-some pounds of higher-functioning substance. Because food makes up a vast majority of the base matter that will be turned into more complex matter (i.e., you as an adult), nutrition should by definition have the capacity to affect a good number of processes. And it does. What one eats has bearing on mood, energy, susceptibility to illness, digestion, sleep, learning, healing capacity, and more. We just do not access nutrition's full healing potential.

WHAT THE SCIENCE SAYS ABOUT NUTRITION

Most people are surprised when they discover how much nutrition affects the everyday health problems all of us face with our children. Does eating a peanut butter sandwich for breakfast rather than a toaster pastry have the power to turn that C in Spanish to a B? Can a child's behavioral problems stem from just being a picky eater? Mom may have told you to eat your vegetables growing up, but how much can eating a few zucchini slices really affect recurring ear infections? The answer is, more than most parents and physicians realize, but not exactly in the way you think.

Most people and most scientific studies look at nutrition in a narrow and reductionist way. People want to see big improvements as a result of one distinct change somehow isolated from the complexity of normal eating and living, while assuming (or pretending) we have correctly identified all the other influencing factors. A classic example of how difficult it is to make any practical decisions with this thinking model is the breakfast studies.

Let's put a very basic nutrition question to the test: Is eating breakfast a good idea? Use your practical experience and answer this question in your mind, because by the time you finish hearing about the scientific studies, you may not even be sure what breakfast is. In science, we need to reduce that question to a narrower concept that can be measured. Therefore, it's not specific enough to ask whether or not eating breakfast is a good idea. We need to know first *who* the potential breakfast eaters are and *what* they are actually eating for breakfast, and then figure out a reliable *measurement* for monitoring the benefits of eating breakfast.

Different studies focus on different aspects of these questions. The focus depends on who is doing the study and, more important, who is paying for it. I like to think of breakfast as the way to jump-start the day by giving your child's body the best possible fuel in the morning when they most need it for energy and learning. My question would be: Will a particular breakfast make your child feel energetic and able to perform well at academic tasks? Let's see what the studies discovered.

One found that eating breakfast regularly significantly reduced stress and depression. That makes sense. It's logical to conclude that starting the day with good food makes a person feel more energetic and better able to cope with stress. But wait . . . The study, funded by

THE NUMBER OF CHILDREN WITH CHRONIC HEALTH CONDITIONS IS INCREASING

According to the American Medical Association, obesity, asthma, behavior and learning problems, and other chronic health conditions increased 14 percent in children between 1994 and 2006. For a health condition to be considered chronic, activities and schooling had to be limited, or medicine, special equipment, or specialized health services had to be required for at least twelve months.

Here are a few more thought-provoking facts from the Centers for Disease Control and Prevention and the U.S. Department of Health and Human Services:

- Five percent of children age five to eleven years missed eleven or more days of school over the last year because of illness or injury.

- Four percent of children under eighteen years of age have food allergies.

- The incidence of food allergies increased 8 percent between 1997 and 2007 in children under age eighteen.

a cereal manufacturer, did not prove that you would be brighter eyed and bushier tailed if you *switched* from not eating breakfast to eating breakfast. The study found only that people who ate any breakfast at all

COULD IT BE HIS DIET?

I realize this list seems long, but all of the issues below can have a nutritional component. If your child is suffering from any of them, examine his diet and consult with a health care practitioner who understands the impact of nutrition on health and well-being.

- autism
- aggression
- allergies
- anxiety
- bad breath
- behavioral issues (including oppositional defiant disorder)
- chewing on clothing or other objects
- clumsiness
- colic
- constipation
- depression
- developmental delays
- diarrhea
- ear infections
- eating disorders
- eczema
- failure to thrive
- frequent illness
- gassiness/bloating
- genital itching (technically known as hands down the pants)
- hives
- hoarse voice
- joint pain
- learning disabilities
- moodiness
- overtiredness
- pica (eating of nonfood items)
- picky eating
- poor healing of wounds
- rashes
- reflux
- seizures
- sensory processing disorder
- sinus infections
- sleep problems
- small stature
- speech delays
- temper tantrums
- tummy aches
- vomiting

tended to feel less stressed and depressed. Maybe, one critic remarked, eating breakfast is just something that happier people do.

If you look at the problem from another angle, you might pose this question: Does it matter if you eat a turkey burger versus a sugary cereal for breakfast? This is a tough, tough question because turkey burger manufacturers have never funded a breakfast study. Cereal manufacturers fund breakfast studies, so the nutrition question has been reduced to whether people who eat Cocoa Puffs versus no breakfast are happier. (Or perhaps happier people eat Cocoa Puffs.)

Certainly, eating breakfast should make students perform better, right? If the child lives in poverty and is malnourished, eating anything in the morning probably makes some difference. But the study results are not as obvious if the child is not starving. Of course, children in higher-income households eat breakfast more often than kids in poorer households and may be getting higher-quality food at other times plus extra tutoring after school, further muddying the breakfast effect. One study discovered that having cereal for breakfast helped school performance compared with having no breakfast. (You can see this one quoted on television commercials, but the results are slightly twisted so that a cereal breakfast appears to be a superior meal rather than just being superior to no food at all.) "There is a lack of research comparing breakfast type, precluding recommendations for the size and composition of an optimal breakfast for children's cognitive function," one researcher lamented. Personally, I am a big fan of eating dinner foods in the morning, but sadly there is no scientific literature documenting the benefits of fish and rice for breakfast.

It turns out that children who eat breakfast tend to be in better nutritional shape to start with and tend to be less overweight. Academic performance definitely goes up when school breakfast programs are put in place, but children also tend to show up for school more often when there is free breakfast, and showing up at school is definitely associated with doing better. The narrow focus of the studies has reduced the application of the results to the funding of school breakfast programs in low-income areas and the marketing of breakfast cereal. Although funding school breakfast programs is a just and worthy cause, none of these studies argues convincingly that a child with access to food would benefit from eating protein for breakfast. We know only that eating breakfast is preferable to being hungry in the morning.

If the most basic nutrition question like this one about breakfast leads to these lackluster findings with limited general application, it's no wonder we lack confidence in our ability to wield the science of nutrition. We constantly give lip service to the idea of diet being important to behavior, growth, and development, but as soon as there is an illness or symptom, medicine is in and nutrition is out. Using a reductionist study model, it's much simpler to test a drug's effectiveness for a certain symptom of disease. Drugs by definition tend to have a specific mode of action, and one pill (versus endless varieties of breakfast, for example) is being studied. Nutrients have a broad spectrum of effects and work in conjunction with other nutrients in a weblike fashion. We know from experience and studies that good nutrition is important for fighting illness, proper growth and development, and optimal learning, but linking one specific condition to one specific nutrient is the exception rather than the rule. Often you are looking at a bigger nutritional picture with several moving parts.

I want to change how we think about chronic conditions, especially those affecting the brain, immune system, and digestive tract. Why not start with the child's personal chemistry, which dictates how his body and brain function? After all, you have enormous influence over the raw materials going into the biochemical soup that is your unique and wonderful child. And, if the first rule of medicine is to do no harm, then the dinner table versus the pharmacy counter is the place to start. What I've studied, witnessed, and tested again and again is that nutrition is a way to tweak a child's personal chemistry for optimal health.

IN A PERFECT WORLD . . .

The foundations of a good diet are simple: whole organic food, lots of fruits and vegetables. Getting this far is already a challenge for most parents because of widespread picky eating problems, which is why the very first nutritional issue to be tackled is the fussy eater. Beyond the basics, most nutritional problems fall into one of two areas: Something being consumed is irritating or something that the body needs is missing. All of the interventions for the health and development problems that follow fall into one of those categories.

In a perfect world, we would not be solving nutrition problems but preventing them. To this end, I am a strong advocate of eating good, healthy food, of course, and also of using nutritional supplements. Supplements close the gap between the ideal and the real, and are insurance against the ravages of modern living. In addition, they can optimize genetic potential in a way that diet alone cannot unless you are willing to make the diet the main focus of your life, and even then, it would be difficult.

One of my dreams is that we as a culture would support healthy eating. In my fantasy utopian nutritional world (cue birds chirping and harp music), farming would make a comeback as a noble and desirable profession.

WHAT DO KIDS REALLY EAT?

According to the Healthy Eating Index-2005, if "good diet" were a class taught at school, most kids would be flunking. The Healthy Eating Index is a measure of diet quality as defined by federal guidelines. The average score for all age groups did not meet the 2005 dietary guidelines for fruits, vegetables, legumes, whole grains, and oils. Unfortunately, children overexcelled in the arena of sodium, bad fats, and added-sugar consumption. An October 2010 study reported that the top sources of calories for two- to eighteen-year-olds were grain desserts (cookies, cakes, granola bars), pizza, and soda. Nearly 40 percent of the total calories consumed were in the form of empty-calorie foods. As horrifying as these statistics were, nobody seemed very surprised by them.

Some of the brightest and most enterprising children when asked what they want to be when they grow up would say proudly, "A farmer." Their adoring parents would beam with the same pride most parents currently reserve for the answers "astronaut" or "investment banker."

I start with a farming renaissance because it is hard to respect the power of food if one does not respect the farmer. In our culture, respect follows income. Therefore farmers would have to make a reasonable living, which means the average person would expect to pay a higher percentage of their income for decent, safe food. The result might mean that we'd have slightly fewer pairs of shoes in our closet and perhaps fewer electronic gadgets, but we'd have more wholesome, organically raised food.

The abundant availability of organically raised food is important because the mass production of cheap, environmentally unconscious food is destroying our land and waterways. In addition, it is subjecting people to the unknown but frightening risk of consuming an untested cocktail of chemicals on a daily basis. The most vulnerable people are children. The skyrocketing number of kids with developmental issues cannot help but make a reasonable person wonder if our unchecked use of preservatives, pesticides, genetically modified foods, additives, colorants, and other substances is contributing to the epidemic.

In my new worldview, chemicals would be tested for safety both alone and in combination with already approved substances before they could be sprayed on crops and used in manufacturing. Currently, they have to be proved harmful before they are banned or regulated, a subtle-sounding but powerful distinction that allows all manner of questionable substance usage. Better to use pesticides and herbicides occasionally when other less environmentally invasive methods fail, the way a pediatrician might use a powerful drug.

Pediatricians, in a nutritionally perfect world, would also be more food-savvy. Instead of one elective course in nutrition, they would be required to take a whole year of nutrition training. Part of that would include a course on how nutrition affects development. As a result, pediatricians would recommend probiotics and fish oil while hesitating to prescribe antibiotics and stimulants except in the most difficult cases.

If a parent complained that three-year-old Amy was a terribly picky eater, the nutritionally aware doctor would have a serious conversation on the benefits of a varied, nutritious diet. They would know better than to brush off the parent with, "Don't worry about it, all kids are picky eaters" or "As long as she is on the growth chart, she is fine." Wouldn't it be nice if the doctor prescribed a few vegetables a day? Parents might feel more confident insisting that their children eat real food.

Instead, the overwhelmed parent is left to walk down the aisles of the supermarket while Amy screams for cookies and crackers. To help the harried parent in my nutritionally perfect world, the sugared cereals and breakfast toaster pastries would be kept behind the pharmacy counter right next to the cold medicines that can be turned into crystal meth. A parent would have to ask for the worthless junk food and would receive a warning notice about the dangers of feeding children these empty non-foods for breakfast. Artificial colors would be removed from all food, or at least foods containing them would include a warning like the one that's now required in the European Union.

Parents would further be supported by a huge government publicity campaign to reduce serving sizes. Teenagers guzzling supersized drinks would be portrayed as "uncool" and, if possible, "un-American." Yes, this sounds a little extreme until one realizes that the opposite is already true. Somewhere along the line "bigger is better" started to be applied to serving size, and America is now associated with supersized portions.

Clearly, we are not living in an ideal nutritional world, so we must labor under the conditions we have. These suboptimal conditions leave you, the parents, caregivers, and mentors of this generation, with a big nutrition job to do.

It is easy to get overwhelmed by all the conflicting and confusing nutrition information being tossed around while trying to navigate a health care system that is stressed to the breaking point. You will need to know how to think

NUTRITION DETECTIVE
PRINCIPLE #1

The Binary Law of Nutrition

All nutritional problems fall into one of two categories: Either something is bothering the body or something is missing. When beginning to solve your child's nutrition conundrum, ask yourself, Do these clues point to an irritant or a deficiency? In other words, is my child reacting to something he is eating or is he not getting enough of something?

When you first ask this question, you may not be able to distinguish between the two, and, to confuse matters, often both problems are present. Not to worry. Your sorting skills will improve as you read more and more examples of each, and if you get stuck with your own child, you can consult an experienced professional. The goal is not to become a nutrition genius yourself, but to know enough to ask the right questions and get the help you need.

15

about nutrition so you can sort through and pick out the relevant information from all the chatter. I will help you become more empowered by teaching you the lesser-known practical uses of therapeutic nutrition and how to apply them. As a result, you will become a better health and nutrition detective so that you can be the best advocate for your own children or any you care about.

Throughout the cases and chapters that follow, you will see that I begin to solve the riddle of any case using this basic but essential question: Is some food bothering the child or is something missing? As you become your child's nutrition detective, you will return to this question again and again.

CHAPTER 2

Becoming a Nutrition Detective

I CALL MYSELF A NUTRITION DETECTIVE because the minute a parent and a child walk into my office, I begin to look for clues. My first step is to listen to their story. I know from many years of experience that parents know a lot about their kids and often are intuitive about the source of a problem. I remember one case very clearly in which a mother "just knew" that her daughter's excessive crying had something to do with the high-fructose corn syrup in the laxative she was prescribed for constipation. She wanted to take her daughter off the medicine but did not want the constipation to return. This mother was right; her daughter was very reactive to corn, and listening to her was the beginning of discovering a better solution for her entire situation.

The next step I take is to examine the child's diet and symptoms for clues: A rash might indicate a sensitivity to dairy products, but it also might indicate an essential fatty acid depletion. A stomachache could mean lactose intolerance, but it might also be caused by a reaction to gluten. Picky eating might be the result of, among other causes, an extreme reaction to the sensory experience of eating food, or it could be caused by a deficiency of the mineral zinc. By paying attention to a child's symptoms and learning to see symptoms or conditions in the context of your child's particular "story," a whole range of strategies present themselves.

You are about to become a nutrition detective. You will learn everything you need to know about decoding your own child's symptoms by reading stories about kids suffering with these familiar and very common childhood issues that nevertheless can have a negative effect on their everyday lives.

Most parents are too busy to sit down and read a dry nutrition book cover to cover. They are also tired of wading through well-meaning advice on how to live with allergies, reflux, and other complicated conditions, or being handed a quick prescription to address symptoms rather than a plan to attack the cause of the problem. By following certain health clues, you will not only become familiar with the information about symptoms, causes, and treatment, but will discover how to become your child's best health advocate, learning how to watch the symptoms, follow the clues,

WE EAT FAST FOOD BECAUSE EVERYONE ELSE DOES

A recent study found that greater exposure to fast food marketing is linked to increased fast food intake among children. Furthermore, the more parents perceived fast food consumption as the social norm, the more frequently their children ate fast food. This was true for everyone in the study, not just members of specific ethnic groups.

Many adults think they are immune to advertising because they are not paying attention to commercials or think ads are stupid. They are wrong. Advertisers study human behavior carefully, specifically using the science and art of persuasion. Research on persuasion consistently finds that people want to be considered "normal." Therefore, the key to effectively selling a new concept begins by defining that which people think of as "normal." By showing continuous images of busy modern families grabbing burgers on the way to soccer practice or eating together at the local fried chicken establishment, the fast food industry has successfully defined the norm and therefore helped pattern our behavior.

and determine what's missing or necessary to avoid. You will learn about how common medicines can interfere with your child's health and often mask the real problem. I have included usable information about vitamins, minerals, and other supplements that can boost your child's mood and her performance and confidence in school, and put her more at ease in social situations. You will learn how to put your detective work into action, determine if an approach is working and when to expect results, and, in some cases, recognize when an approach may not be working, so that you can make an educated change in treatment. For parents interested in sharing information with their doctors or getting more details, there are references to scientific studies and suggestions for further reading at the end of the book.

Again, some of these strategies do take some trial and error as you watch and wait for your child to respond. But the goal is for you to be able to use what you learn to resolve intrusive, painful physical symptoms to increase your child's sense of well-being, confidence, and ease in his own body.

THINKING LIKE A DETECTIVE

To figure out if your child's problem has a nutritional cause, you have to start thinking like a detective. A great detective has to observe, analyze, and be curious. Rudyard Kipling called this point of view "insatiable curiosity" in his short story about an elephant child. I believe this is the most important characteristic of an effective detective. Ask questions about everything. Talk to other parents about their kids' habits and health and see how they relate to your child's. How did they respond to the symptoms? What did they do to intervene? Did they consult an expert beyond their pediatrician? Who was it and what did that person do? What characteristics does this child share with your offspring?

Becoming a good nutrition detective means paying attention to your gut and learning to trust it, as well as drawing on information you may have read or heard. There is no irrelevant learning to a detective: Every detail can play a role in solving the problem or cause behind your child's illness. Many parents are not aware of how much they know, or think their own "gut feelings" are not important or accurate. Often parents will say, "I read that . . ." or "I heard that . . ." Parents pay a lot of attention to what they read when it comes to nutrition and their children, but there has been no single place to connect all the dots and understand how seemingly arcane or unrelated facts apply to our own health situations. Many of the parents with whom I work simply

> Many parents are not aware of how much they know, or think their own "gut feelings" are not important or accurate.

don't know how to turn their observations and knowledge into usable information to help their children.

Let's build your confidence by confirming what you might already suspect while filling in with lots of interesting bits of data needed to make the whole puzzle come together. You certainly do not have to remember all the details, but once you know about the possibilities, your thinking will be forever changed. This is how nutrition-detective thinking works.

A recent case shows this step-by-step process in action. I was in Chicago, teaching an all-day course on children's development and nutrition. The hotel ballroom was packed with interesting people with endless questions. After eight hours, I was cursing the person who had thought up the "all-day" course. Did she have feet? I wondered irritably. As I packed up my computer, one last straggler, a woman in her early thirties, approached me. "May I talk to you for a few minutes?" she asked nervously.

The woman was dressed casually and looked pleasant enough, but I noticed that she was wringing her hands. Before I could say, "Of course," her story started pouring out. She did not know where to turn. Ever since her baby had been born (eight months earlier) the poor woman had been miserable. At first, she thought her exhaustion was caused by having a new baby and not getting enough sleep, but then the joint pain started. Her doctor discovered she had Lyme disease and prescribed a course of antibiotics, but after weeks of taking them, she didn't feel any better.

The story continued on and on, and my brain was getting tired trying to follow all of the details. The woman went to see another doctor, who prescribed more antibiotics and more tests, but to no avail—the new mother again did not improve. Her most recent blood test had still been positive for Lyme.

There were probably more important clues in her painful story, but I could barely follow the conversation, let alone sort the details. Many parents are in this exact situation with their own child's story. They are overwhelmed, exhausted, and emotionally unable to figure out what the situation means. A good parent perseveres, and the least I could do was the same.

The first step when a problem is overwhelming is to strip it down to the bare facts. Removing the emotional components or confusing side stories can help clarify the situation. My fuzzy mind picked out the following basic facts:

- exhaustion
- Lyme disease that is not responding to antibiotics
- joint pain
- new mother

In medicine, there might be ten common conditions with this group of symptoms. Much of early medical training involves learning about large numbers of conditions and their accompanying set of symptoms. Then, when a patient presents with a specific group of complaints, the well-trained physician can identify the ailment. Any group of symptoms will have a small or large group of possible explanations, and the doctor will work through his mental list of possible causes until he more or less matches the patient's symptoms with a diagnosis. As in all detective work, some of these facts may not be relevant to the primary problem and the critical fact may be missing. In other words, we don't always know what we don't know, in which case, even a very good doctor might come to an inaccurate conclusion or diagnosis.

Everyone has suffered and then been blindsided because they did not know enough to consider a piece of information critical. Recently a mother brought her developmentally delayed six-year-old to see me. His language skills were so far behind those of his peers that he could not make friends or be placed in a regular classroom. I outlined a detailed plan for how to support the biochemistry of learning and what she could do that might help him catch up. Toward the end of the session I could see she was becoming very emotional.

"Is everything all right?" I asked with concern. "Are you comfortable with this plan?"

"I am so upset that I did not come and see you when I first got your name two years ago," she confessed. When asked what stopped her she said, "I just could not imagine how nutrition would help. My doctor said it was probably a waste of time, so I concentrated on other therapies." How many average mothers know to consider the biochemistry of learning when faced with a developmental delay? Not many. She thought she was doing all she could, and she had been doing all she could with the information she had at the time.

WHAT AN AVERAGE DOCTOR CAN BE EXPECTED TO KNOW

In addition to the ten possible common conditions associated with any ailment list, there could be as many as fifty strange and unusual conditions that only a handful of specialists are trained to recognize or consider. Diagnosing a rare condition can take years, because you have to run into a doctor who has heard of or has experience with the "odd stuff." Rare conditions are called rare for a reason. Sherlock Holmes was considered a detective genius because of his near-encyclopedic knowledge of arcane and rare bits of information that could take otherwise meaningless clues and piece them together. "I noticed, dear Watson, that the victim had a distinct pink tinge. Clearly, that indicated he was mercury poisoned, so I knew I had to look in . . ." and so on. The pink coloring has meaning only if one already knows it is a sign of mercury toxicity (which it is). This is a character in literature, not a model for the perfect pediatrician.

Of the hypothetical list of ten common causes, how many can the average doctor be expected to identify? According to Dr. Lisa Sanders, author of the book *Every Patient Tells a Story,* studies find the average doctor is sorely lacking physical exam skills. Dr. Sanders is the medical consultant for a TV medical show, *House,* in which the doctor not only always knows all ten common possibilities but is an expert on the fifty weird conditions associated with every symptom list, too. In real life, Dr. Sanders reports that when evaluating cardiac exam skills, graduating medical students correctly answered just over half the questions. Their teacher-physicians and doctors in practice did a little better, correctly answering almost 60 percent of the questions. If these questions are a test of cardiac exam skills, the grade for the average doctor is 50 to 60 percent, or failing. She quotes further studies that found that doctors and patients disagreed about the main reason for a patient's visit, otherwise known as the chief complaint, 25 to 50 percent of the time. One can therefore expect that in the average visit to a regular doctor, half the time she will not know why you are there or what she is looking at.

What is the significance of this study? It does not mean that physicians are poorly trained or that they don't know their jobs; what it does suggest is that physicians have human brains capable of holding only so much information at any one time. The same is true of plumbers, actors, and even nutritionists. A gigantic database is needed to consider every possibility, and we all have a finite amount of facts and experiences at our disposal (i.e., in our recall memory) at any given time.

The reason people sometimes need to see four, five, or ten medical professionals for some complaints is to cover a wider base of possibilities. Because it is impossible to remember or have experience with all causative factors, all professionals tend to concentrate on and emphasize certain ones. In general, doctors tend to diagnose the most common conditions they were trained to find with clear, agreed-upon diagnostic criteria.

The fact remains that nutritional conditions and factors are not generally part of most doctors' medical training or experience base, so patients have to develop their own information base or look outside regular channels. Rather than expect doctors to know how to do gastric surgery *and* recall which foods contain folic acid, today's medical consumers have to know more and help medical professionals help them.

This is where you, the parent, come in. You have to keep the professionals you consult on task and make sure they are clear about why you are seeking their advice. Start by keeping an accurate record of when your child's symptoms began, changed (got worse or better), and any other factors that may seem the least bit relevant to you.

You also should remember to help the doctor or health care provider keep the facts straight, especially if the case is complex. I recommend that parents keep a notebook or file for all health incidents, questions, or any observation that seems significant. Do not expect them to be TV doctors or computers with a bottomless medical database. To be successful, you will have to be an active part of the team.

RULING OUT SUSPECTS

Now back to the distraught new mother at the conference. Given the number of doctors the woman had seen, I assumed the common medical suspects were ruled out and she was fishing in the "rare" pool. Was there anything in my experience in the nutrition world that could shed light on her situation? The doctors had been thorough and she had been given a diagnosis (Lyme disease), which was supported by blood work.

I considered a few clues: Several antibiotics had been tried, so the disease could be antibiotic resistant. Antibiotic resistance is a common, frightening problem beyond my abilities to correct, so I put it aside for the moment.

I then explored the possible nutritional reasons why the treatment was not working. What in the diet interferes with antibiotics? Usually, it is antibiotics interfering with other medicines, such as birth control pills, or causing trouble with the good bacteria while killing the bad. Does anything prey on antibiotics?

There is one mineral that not only stops antibiotics from working but can interfere with immune response. That mineral is iron. Bacteria thrive on iron and cannot grow without it.

The woman was a new mother. In my experience, new mothers often continue taking prenatal vitamins either because they are convenient or because they are thinking of getting pregnant again. Prenatal vitamins contain extra-high amounts of iron.

"Are you still taking your prenatal vitamins?" I asked.

"Yes, I had them so I just kept taking them," she confirmed.

Bingo.

I now had a possible explanation for her problems. Prenatal vitamins contain much higher levels of iron than traditional women's vitamins. Bacteria love iron, and Lyme disease is caused by a group of bacteria. Scientists have long known that when bacteria are grown in a petri dish and the right antibiotic is added, the bacteria die. However, if iron is also added, the bacteria survive in spite of the antibiotics. Further, when the body is developing an infection, levels of a protein called lactoferrin start to increase dramatically. The job of lactoferrin is to bind up as much iron as possible so the bacteria cannot feed on it. I told the distraught woman to call her doctor immediately and tell her about the probable though unintended effect of her prenatal vitamin.

THE SEVEN QUESTIONS EVERY NUTRITION DETECTIVE MUST ASK

Stripping the story down to its bare facts is an excellent starting place to figuring out how to begin your investigation into what's ailing your child, especially when you are emotionally involved or overwhelmed by a situation. Finding the bones of a story is what I do when the amount of information someone is providing is excessive or they are distraught and discombobulated. It does not take into account the complex emotional and social factors surrounding the issues, but the technique helps organize your thinking. There are seven essential questions that you will ask about your child any time you are trying to discover if his or her symptoms might have a nutritional cause and solution.

1. What are the facts? Take a few minutes to jot down as many facts and thoughts as you can about your child's concern, including any previous illnesses or events that might be related or might have led up to the present situation. Bullet or number the information rather than writing a narrative. Some people use an old calendar and fill in the history on it.

2. Which symptoms worry you the most?

3. When did the symptoms start?

4. Do the symptoms come and go? Have they changed over time?

5. What else was going on in your child's life when the symptoms started? If your child is five or younger, any health condition can be related to or affect development. Perhaps at the same time that you noticed skin rashes, your eleven-month-old was just starting to walk and had recently had a few ear infections. Or you noticed that your five-year-old seemed more distracted after he had the flu.

6. What was your child's diet when the symptoms started?

7. Was your child on any medications? When did they start and stop?

If you have any theories or have received any advice, jot that down separately. Initially, write down exactly what happened on one list (just the facts) and your ideas about why on another. That way, your assessment of the information will not color the story from the beginning and prevent you from considering all interpretations. As you assemble this record of your child's symptoms, you begin to create his or her health "story," which will help you communicate this information to a doctor, nutritionist, or other health care provider if necessary.

HIDING IN PLAIN SIGHT

I helped Lily with her son Milo's story. Lily entered my office after a three-year absence. She had first come to see me about her eldest son, Charlie. Charlie had frequent ear and upper respiratory infections, which had been so bad that they were interfering with his speech development. The problems started when Lily stopped nursing him and he started on whole milk at age one. We decided his immune issues might stem from reactions to dairy protein and had taken him off all cow's milk products. Lily had been reluctant to implement a dairy-free trial because Charlie loved his bottle and little else. It took a few sessions with me providing supporting evidence, cajoling, and practically begging until she finally agreed to remove dairy from his diet.

Within weeks Charlie was dramatically better and back on a normal developmental curve. We increased his calcium intake to support his bones and teeth, and I did not hear from the family again. But now, she was back to talk about her younger son, Milo, now a toddler.

I pulled out Charlie's old notes, just in case she wanted to ask me a question about him. During the initial pleasantries, Lily reported that Charlie was doing great and was as healthy as a horse. Still, patterns can occur in families, and at the time, I could not remember the details of what had happened three years earlier.

"Milo is always sick," she began. "At two, he picks up every cough or cold going around. He's also had at least four ear infections." At first, Lily thought Charlie was bringing home bugs from school, but she realized Charlie was no longer sick very often. Milo was a picky eater, preferring to drink milk from his bottle.

My eyes were darting back and forth. Did this not sound familiar to her? I could just reread Charlie's old notes and know the rest of the story.

Lily is a well-educated, intelligent woman. Why was she spending money to come back and see me when she could just take Milo off dairy like his brother?

I wanted to help her find the answer for herself, because she already knew the solution to her "new" problem. Stripping down the story, I told her almost the same fact pattern she had told me three years earlier. There was a small difference, with Milo tending more toward sinus infections, whereas Charlie had tended to get bronchitis. Both brothers were sick frequently and had ear infections.

"Yes," she said, nodding in agreement. "You have it."

"What do you think it is?" I prompted.

"I really don't know," she fretted. Here is where the emotional part comes in and why we need help when thinking about our own children.

"Does this story ring any bells?" I shamelessly hinted.

"No," she insisted, but now she was fidgeting.

"This is Charlie's story all over again," I said as gently as I could. "You must have noticed the similarities."

"Well, of course I thought about it," she sighed miserably, "but I really, really did not want to have to do the no-dairy thing again."

"But you are still doing it for Charlie. What is the big deal?" I persisted.

"Well, I was hoping something else could be going on," she admitted. "But if not, I am here so you can talk me into it."

Parents often suspect the answer, but when it comes to their children and eating, they can get stuck in their thinking. Lily's instincts were right on. She knew there was a nutritional problem but did not want to go through the same process she had with her older son without someone confirming her suspicions. She told me exactly what she needed: a knowledgeable person to agree with her or, as she said, talk her into it. All I had to do was nod my head in agreement and remind her what she already knew.

Often parents suspect they need to follow a course of action, but when they do not want to, the whole situation suddenly seems confusing and unclear. Certain foods can have emotional meaning, and taking away foods can be difficult. Some parents worry that kids will stop eating altogether. Both Charlie and Milo were huge milk guzzlers, and Lily understandably wondered how her fussy eaters were going to make up for all those calories. She had successfully transitioned Charlie to other healthy foods, but as a busy mother of two it was just easier to hand Milo a bottle, which he loved. Lily had worked out the story weeks ago but not her feelings. Luckily, she knew what kind of help she needed to get unstuck.

Again, it's important that you get clear on your child's story, because you will feel much more confident trusting your own instincts about what's going on with your child. Then use the seven questions to fill in the information you need to make the facts make sense as you begin to assemble the other clues. In the next few chapters you will see how different cases were solved, nutrition-style. No doubt you will begin to see clues and patterns emerge. At first, you might not know what the clues mean, but as you progress and become more and more familiar with nutritional thinking and knowledge, you will not only begin thinking like a detective but feel more confident about what kind of help your child needs.

OBESITY: A NUTRITIONAL OR CULTURAL PROBLEM?

In the early years, I believed the powers of nutrition were endless. There was no problem that good nutrition could not improve. Of course, there turned out to be plenty of limitations. The most disappointing results occurred with the very condition I was taught nutrition could cure: obesity. Time after time I was frustrated to find that the right nutrition program did not cure obesity. Dozens of diets and lifestyle changes worked, but most people would not or could not stick with them. Statistics I uncovered suggested that the number of people who permanently maintain weight loss hovers around a dismal 10 percent.

Results from weight loss programs are so poor that insurance companies cite them as an excuse not to cover obesity treatment (except for surgery). There were many other issues involved in why people were inclined to overeat and unable to maintain weight loss, including social pressure, poor self-esteem, time constraints, feelings of deprivation, unconsciousness around eating, and addiction—all highlighting the limitations of diet alone.

Helping overweight and obese children was even worse. The parents did not want their children to be overweight, but understandably, they were unable to deprive their children, who were, they argued, hungry or being left out of social events. Or, the mothers worried they would create an eating disorder or poor self-esteem by addressing dietary problems. Often the parents were overweight and could not do for their child what they could not do for themselves.

The experts at esteemed institutions are doing no better with our chubby children. In some cases, they are contributing to the problem. One not-to-be-named well-known hospital advises parents not to overly restrict sugar consumption in their diabetic teenagers because it is "too hard on them" and they need to "feel normal." Instead, parents are told to increase the amount of insulin prescribed to balance the extra sugar. The result of increasing insulin to metabolize sugar in a diabetic is predictable and unavoidable weight gain.

I have concluded that obesity is not a nutritional problem but a cultural one. Our entire culture conspires against weight loss, and this thorny issue will not be solved by nutritionists. For this reason, you will not find a chapter in this book on childhood obesity. Our wonderful intellectual solutions don't work at all. Although I concede temporary defeat in this area, I am hopeful we will one day take on this problem as a culture.

In the meantime, there are plenty of other nutritional battles you can fight, and win. My nutrition philosophy is optimistic but also realistic. I understand that all medical problems have a number of contributing factors and nutrition is but one of many, but wait until you see what is possible.

SHARING INFORMATION WITH YOUR DOCTOR

The first concept a good psychotherapist tries to convey when beginning therapy is that no one can change another person. This is useful information, whether you're frustrated with your spouse, boss, or doctor. If your pediatrician or specialist is not interested in your input or has strong personal views about nutrition, no amount of wishing they were different will change them. You will make them angry and yourself frustrated by trying. Early in my career I would send research articles and educational materials to doubting health care professionals, and inevitably even the most compelling, scientifically valid information would not sway a made-up mind. The research studies were not done by the "right" people or were not good enough. Several times professionals said

> When you're visiting a doctor, prioritize your concerns and address one or two (maximum) issues.

with unabashed haughtiness that if the idea were so useful, they would have known about it before. These rigid thinkers require a huge personal crisis or an act of God to shift their thinking. In other words, not me or you.

As you begin this process of getting involved in your child's nutrition, it's key to find a professional who is more interested in your child's health than in being right. You also want to find out if he or she is open-minded and flexible. Luckily, there are many wonderful professionals with these characteristics. Unfortunately, they sometimes have long waiting lists when you do find them.

Once you find a doctor who is supportive of and knowledgeable about nutrition, try to avoid overwhelming him or her with huge amounts of information. Copy a chapter or send over this book with the most relevant part marked. Or find a study abstract or a short, to-the-point synopsis highlighting your question or concern. Prioritize your concerns and address one or two (maximum) issues in a visit. Most office visits

31

Children act bad when they feel bad.

Of course, there are a hundred reasons kids can feel bad. Depending on their age and the nature of the problem, youngsters can have difficulty pinpointing an area of discomfort. One well-known gastrointestinal specialist once remarked that until age twelve, children could not consistently give him accurate information so he could diagnose their conditions. The universal language for children is their behavior. So my advice is this: If your child is acting bad or in a way that is not typical, follow the clues. He may indeed be responding to a physiological problem that he is otherwise unable to describe to you.

are not long enough for more processing. If you try to deal with more, the doctor, not you, will be forced to pick what gets covered.

The average visit to a doctor's office lasts about fifteen minutes. What are the chances of thoroughly covering three areas of concern in that amount of time? None. In addition, your doctor is not a trained psychologist or talk therapist. If you start talking about how you are worried about this and concerned about that, he will be doing triage in his head, listening for the most significant and serious symptoms and addressing them, ideally within the allowed time. He will interrupt you, often within the first twenty seconds, according to studies, and direct you toward the information he thinks he needs to solve the most pressing concerns. That is what he is trained to do.

There are wonderful doctors who spend much more time with their patients and help them sort out large amounts of confusing information and test results. Expect them to be more expensive and not covered by insurance. One such doctor is Neil Spiegel, a physiatrist who trained at the New York University Rusk Institute of Rehabilitation Medicine. As a specialist in physical medicine and rehabilitation, he mostly deals with patients who are experiencing chronic pain. Because pain conditions are complex, he did extra training in nutrition, physical therapy, acupuncture, and psychology, and just for fun, earned a master's degree in business—all so he could be as effective as possible when trying to ease the pain of suffering patients. I asked him how he integrates nutrition into his work.

"A nine-year-old elite soccer player was brought in by his parents," Dr. Spiegel explained, setting up his example.

"A nine-year-old elite soccer player," I snorted in disbelief. "Starting early for the Olympics?"

"That was his parents' plan," Dr. Spiegel continued, unfazed. The problem was that Trey, the child, kept getting hurt and was not healing. The most persistent injury was a recurrent groin strain, but he also had frequent nosebleeds and stomach pain. Dr. Spiegel had done a physical exam, taught Trey some proper stretching exercises, and run some basic blood tests to rule out autoimmune disease and inflammatory conditions. All the tests came back normal, and unfortunately the stretching didn't help Trey.

Using his psychology training, Dr. Spiegel surreptitiously questioned Trey about his desire to play soccer. Maybe Trey secretly did not like soccer but was playing to satisfy his ambitious parents. Dr. Spiegel asked Trey, "Do you look forward to your games? What do you like about playing?"

Trey responded flatly but honestly, "Yes" and "I'm not sure." Alas, there was no gold to mine there.

Next, Dr. Spiegel pulled out the acupuncture needles. Acupuncture treatment helped the injuries heal faster, but Trey kept getting them, and the nosebleeds did not improve.

"There are a couple of reasons why people have nosebleeds—picking your nose, for example. Do you do that?" Dr. Spiegel asked Trey.

"Sometimes," Trey responded.

The direction of the conversation got Dr. Spiegel thinking. Using his acupuncture training, he recognized a connection between the stomach and nose. The stomach and nose are also connected in Western medicine, because there is a tube that starts in the nose, passes through the esophagus, and becomes the stomach. Via these connections, something bothering your stomach can affect your nose.

"Things don't just happen—they happen for a reason," Dr. Spiegel was explaining to me. "They have to be connected."

What bothers the stomach is usually food, so he looked at Trey's diet. There were many bagels and sandwiches, and there was lots of pasta. All of these items are made from wheat and contain the wheat protein gluten, which when not tolerated causes stomach pain and can cause healing issues. He recommended a gluten-free diet for Trey.

Trey's blood screening for celiac disease (an autoimmune disease triggered by eating gluten) came out normal, but once he was off gluten, all his symptoms disappeared within a few weeks. When he cheated a couple of times, the stomachaches and nosebleeds came back immediately, so he stopped before the injuries could start.

Dr. Spiegel is a talented nutrition detective. You, too, can hone your sleuthing skills by asking lots of questions, trusting your instincts, if necessary recognizing that you may not be asking the right questions (for example, if the situation is not improving), and optimizing your time with medical professionals.

As we move forward, you will discover that nutrition can be helpful in ways you have never considered.

CHAPTER 3

The Conundrum of Picky Eating

O NE OF THE MOST COMMON QUESTIONS I receive from parents is what to do about their picky eater. They usually have talked to their pediatrician and been assured all is well, but they worry nonetheless. Most doctors will tell you that when children are picky eaters but are otherwise healthy—meaning they are on the growth chart in terms of height and weight and are not anemic—"they're fine." And although some kids do outgrow picky eating, slowly but surely adding more variety to their diet as they get older, many others need help.

Should you be worried if you have a picky eater? Absolutely not. Worrying is bad for your health. But it is an important internal nudge to look more closely at what may be going on underneath your child's pickiness. In fact, your concern is your inner detective sensing something amiss. Acknowledge the worry, gather information, and make a plan. A child who restricts herself to eating an empty-calorie, low-nutrient diet (often made up of pasta, bread, cheese, french fries, sweets, and other bland comfort foods) is not getting enough nutrients to

OUR PICKY GENERATION

The American Heart Association recommends feeding children a fruit or vegetable with every meal. By age fourteen, the organization recommends 3 cups of vegetables per day for future heart health. Most nutritional professionals generally recommend that children eat four to five servings of fruits and vegetables (not just fruit) per day. Only about 20 percent of children in the United States are meeting this standard. Canada is just as bad, with only about 14 percent of children between nine and twelve meeting these dietary goals, according to the Canadian Community Health Survey. About a quarter of those few vegetables are french fries. No wonder the common wisdom is that picky eating is the norm. Common, yes; good, no—especially when what kids are eating instead are snack foods and soda. And everybody (except possibly candy manufacturers) agrees that this trend is making kids fatter and setting them up for future disease.

grow and develop optimally. Because these kids rely on high-starch, high-fat foods that often lack essential nutrients and the bonus healing substances found in fruits, vegetables, fish, and whole grains, they can tend toward moodiness, irritability, and fatigue . . . just like adults who eat poorly. Also, they can become easily overwhelmed, sleep poorly, and not perform up to their physical or academic potential. Think of it this way: The body is not the government—it cannot run effectively or efficiently on a deficit.

Picky eating can make kids tired and irritable, but it can also be a sign of underlying medical issues such as reflux and colon impaction. Vibrant children have healthy appetites. And finally, kids who are picky eaters are just darn stressful to feed. They can turn dinner into a horrible experience for the whole family, making everybody involved dread mealtimes. It's challenging enough for most of us to make dinner at the end of the day, never mind the Herculean effort of dealing with an exhausted and cranky kid who requires a separate meal, constant cajoling, and ongoing negotiating, with many a night ending in angry outbursts and tears (usually shed by the parents at this point).

If you are living with a picky eater, you are probably recalling some of those not-so-precious mealtime moments right now. In a desperate attempt to be a good parent and have her eat something—anything—healthy, you may have yelled things at your child that you would not confess to your priest. You are not alone, and neither is your child. All picky eaters have unique characteristics that can be rooted in multiple causes, some of which may be physical or medical in nature, others of which might be more emotional or behavioral, or a mix of the two. For that reason, when it comes to picky eating, each case needs to be figured out individually and in the context of that child's "story." That said, let me share a case that is quite typical and will show how you can follow the clues (i.e., the myriad symptoms) that unlock the mystery (i.e., the multiple causes) behind the picky eating and show you what you can do. In the next chapter, you will learn about my E.A.T. program, which can help all parents whose kids have diets that are too limited. Even if your child is not "ill," a poor diet may be limiting his or her full health and academic potential.

THE MANY MOODS OF TOM

Tom was four years old when his pediatrician sent him to me. The first thing I noticed about him was that he did not look healthy. His skin was the color of paste, accented by dark circles under his eyes. His mother told me that he was a very sensitive boy who cried easily, had a hard time with transitions, and found it difficult to play with other children. I also learned that when he was younger, he was sick a lot with many upper respiratory infections and had so many ear infections that he had had tubes put in at eighteen months. At four, he was sleeping poorly almost every night and was continually cranky. Although his pediatrician could not find any specific medical problem, she finally agreed with Tom's mother that there must be some reason behind his sallow complexion and general grumpiness. Maybe a nutritionist would help.

Within a few minutes of talking to Tom's mother, it was apparent that Tom was famous in the family for his picky eating. (His older brother

CAN PICKY EATING AFFECT IQ?

Twins are favorite subjects among researchers because, in theory, they present a way to test and isolate the influence of nurture on nature. Identical twins raised together can provide a similar environment for testing a single factor, and those raised apart can test the effect of environment on genetic predisposition. The single factor of picky eating was studied in identical twins (raised together), in which one sibling was a good eater and the other picky. Even subtle differences in eating behavior between twins caused small but reliable discrepancies in mental development, especially in verbal scores. The picky eaters consistently did worse across the board as they developed and performed in school. Because they had the same genes, differences in performance could not be attributed to differing genetic predisposition. More disturbing, boys were more affected than girls.

The authors made this bold statement: "The data relating early feeding problems with later mental abilities suggest a caution to those responsible for the care of young children, i.e., that 'picky eating,' chronic 'spitting up,' colic, or refusal of classes of foods should not be taken too lightly." In other words, picky eating is not a passing phase to be ignored, and nor should one accept such conditions as colic and reflux as a given for newborns, babies, or toddlers.

had held the title until Tom came along.) If his mother could even get him to sit down and eat, he would take a couple of bites and then push his plate away. He seemed to be surviving on pancakes, grilled cheese, ice cream, milk, cookies, and endless crackers.

Tom's mother was a speech pathologist and knew a lot about child development. She was convinced something significant was afoot and had consequently taken Tom to a number of specialists, including a neurologist, an orthopedist, a physical therapist, a developmental pediatrician, and another speech therapist. She recognized that he was a terrible eater, but what drove her to get nutrition help was her son's mood and behavior, which swung from wonderful to evil in a nanosecond throughout much of the day. (One doctor thought his sleep was so poor that he recommended a sleep study, which did not find any medical issues.) Despite his symptoms, none of these specialists, including teachers and counselors at his school, had found anything specifically "wrong" with Tom.

Nothing in Tom's early childhood pointed to an explanation of the problem, including the fact that his mother had been put on bed rest for the last thirteen weeks of her pregnancy. His twin, a girl, was completely different, healthy in all ways, showing no signs of picky eating. However, Tom's older brother was also a picky eater, and had recently been diagnosed with esophageal reflux. Although he was much happier once the reflux was treated, he still ate a limited diet.

Tom was in bad shape, and we all knew that if nutrition couldn't help, the next step was a psychiatrist, and everyone involved wanted to prevent that if possible.

Tom's mood reactions were demonstrations that his neurological system was out of balance. If a child's neural network is lacking nutrients, it cannot be expected to work optimally. If the components are not there when they are needed, a weaker system is built, and the person compensates accordingly. For example, if a child consumes the wrong kind of fat (the fat that comes from mac-and-cheese, chips, or fried foods instead of fish, whole grains, and lean meats), the cells incorporate the less suitable fat into the membrane. The nerve membrane now is less able to process and interpret incoming signals, resulting in changes in sensory system capabilities. Multiply this problem with foods devoid of nutrients (read: sugar, sugar, sugar!), and a child will be functioning—emotionally, mentally, and physically—at a deficit.

LOOKING FOR CLUES

Not all picky eaters are created equal. As your child's nutrition detective, it's up to you to follow the clues your child is presenting so you can figure out, along with your health care provider, just what to do. Using Tom as a test case, you can become familiar with the most common symptoms and causes behind picky eating. Does Tom simply have a behavioral problem, or do you have a theory about what else might be happening?

By following the clues that Tom presented, you can become more familiar with this detective process:

1. The first clue is that Tom looked unhealthy and had a history of getting sick frequently. Remember the pasty pallor and dark circles under his eyes? Of course, his mother had always felt that this was a sign that something was wrong, and she was right. But it's very easy for parents to disregard their gut instinct about their child, especially when we're being advised by so many experts! The fact that Tom was frequently sick (colds, ear infections, stomach viruses, throat infections, pneumonia) meant that his immune system was either weak or under assault.

2. The second clue was the fact that none of the five medical specialists Tom had seen had found a single medical explanation for his sleep problems, irritability, or frequent illnesses—never mind the picky eating.

3. The third clue was the fact that Tom's twin was fine, showing none of the same symptoms as Tom. She was being raised in the same environment but ate better. Could it be the eating?

4. A fourth clue was the crazy mood swings. Tom was a fun kid one minute and an impossible tyrant the next. If you can be balanced and happy some of the time, the capacity for being so is there. A child who feels bad often acts bad. Children do not have as strong a capacity for regulating their emotions and reactions as adults.

5. A final clue was Tom's difficulty sleeping. There are a number of possible causes for this, but it was consistent with the rest of his profile: Why should Tom be peaceful at night when he was a mess most of the day? Whatever was bothering him was following him into the night.

WHAT THE CLUES MEAN

Aside from the fact that Tom himself often seemed irritable, many of the clues pointed to irritation as the overarching cause of many of his

THE BINARY LAW OF NUTRITION: A REMINDER

As mentioned in chapter 1, all nutritional problems fall into one of two categories: Either something is bothering the body or something it needs is missing. When beginning to solve your child's nutrition conundrum, always ask yourself these questions: Do these clues point to an irritant or a deficiency? Is my child reacting to something he is eating or is he not getting enough of something?

Irritants are irritating, so some of the symptoms to expect are irritated skin (rashes), an irritated nervous system (trouble sleeping or crankiness), and an irritated digestive system (gas, bloat, constipation, reflux). The tricky part is that sometimes the symptom of a deficiency can present as irritability. One symptom of low blood sugar, for example, is crankiness or irritability, and the solution is to eat blood sugar–stabilizing foods, such as meat, beans, nuts, and whole grains, more regularly. But some irritants, such as corn syrup, cause grogginess or sleepiness whenever consumed. In complicated cases usually both things are happening together. Hint: Tom is complicated.

symptoms. The first important clue was the fact that he was constantly sick. The second was that he could not sleep. Put together crankiness, poor sleep, and frequent illness, throw in a pasty complexion, and the usual suspect is intolerance of dairy protein. The other two common symptoms of dairy protein intolerance that Tom did not have are constipation and skin rashes. Few people have every symptom of intolerance, so the fact that Tom did not have bowel issues or eczema is insignificant.

About 80 percent of the protein in milk is casein, a complicated protein that is difficult for many people to digest. When you think about it, cow's milk is designed for a regurgitant with four stomach chambers. A regurgitant is an animal that "regurgitates" its lunch back into its mouth so it can be rechewed and then swallowed into another chamber. It is a great digestive trick for cows (and possibly some of the thinner movie stars), but most of us cannot do this. Instead, the response to this complicated protein in those who cannot tolerate it is irritation. The body tries to soothe the assault by producing mucus.

41

How does your nose get stuffed up with mucus when the milk is in your stomach? The nose is the beginning outer opening of a long tube. The front end is branched between the nose and the mouth. Then the tube continues down your throat, through the stomach and intestines, and out the backside. If something bothers the tube in one place and there is a mucus response, there can be mucus anywhere along the tube.

If mucus is produced in response to dairy consumption, the body has the perfect breeding ground for bacteria and viruses. All you need are a few germs, and germs are pretty much everywhere. Generally they do not bother you, but if you offer them a welcoming growth medium, poor sleeping patterns, and a lousy diet, throw in a couple of well-placed sneezes or some snotty toys lying on the floor at school, and voilà, another illness.

> An allergic reaction is narrowly defined as symptoms following a histamine response.

Is Tom allergic to dairy? No. An allergic reaction is narrowly defined as symptoms following a histamine response. Histamine causes itching and swelling, and Tom did not have these symptoms. Therefore, allergy testing would not have found the source of his problem. Food reactions and sensitivities are a broader group of responses that are induced by a complicated group of non-histamine messenger chemicals. The wide range of reactions can be anything from joint pain to moodiness. For more about the difference between allergies and reactions/sensitivities, read chapter 5.

When you're stuffy and your entire digestive and respiratory systems are lined with mucus, food doesn't smell or taste good. Of course you don't feel like eating. I was beginning to suspect that Tom's pickiness was more accurately a disinterest in food. If his entire system was coated with a nice layer of phlegm, why would he want to eat?

My first suggestion to Tom's mother was to take dairy completely out of his diet, give him a calcium and multivitamin supplement, and come back and see me in six weeks. I didn't bother to suggest nondairy

WHY YOU SHOULD CARE ABOUT PHYTONUTRIENTS

The word *phytonutrients* literally means "plant nutrients." Thousands of them have been identified in fruits, vegetables, and whole grains. They are not vitamins or minerals and do not have calories, but they are chemicals that may have health benefits. Phytochemicals are broken into classes according to their function in the plant. They are responsible for the color, smell, and taste of foods. Carotenoids, for example, add color to red peppers, tomatoes, carrots, and watermelon, and allylic sulfides give garlic and onions their pungent taste and smell.

The same chemicals that impart taste and smell can also have properties that prevent cancer and reduce inflammation. Broccoli contains a phytonutrient called sulforaphane that researchers have discovered interferes with tumor growth and may reduce the risk of breast cancer. Therefore, the most important reason for eating broccoli may not be the identified essential nutrients, such as vitamin A, but the substances that make it tangy and green that while important have not yet been identified as essential.

---

alternatives to cheese or milk. Although there are many such products, they rarely pass the kid taste test, and their nutritional value is limited (rice milk, for example). In addition, it's been my experience that kids who go off dairy acclimate in time (how long this takes varies) and naturally begin to include other protein sources, including meat, beans, peanut or other nut butters, and even hearty grains with higher protein.

Tom's mother called me the next week to say that his appetite had increased almost immediately and that he had begun eating a lot more red meat and chicken. (Meat and chicken offer a high concentration of protein, vitamins, and minerals in general.) The other almost immediate change was that Tom began to sleep much better and became a lot calmer, with far fewer outbursts. These two responses to taking the dairy out indicated that dairy had indeed been an irritant for Tom.

As you will see in the cases ahead, there can often be a bit more trial and error to discover an irritant in disguise, and at other times, you may discover that a child is not reacting to an irritant but responding to a lack of some kind of nutrient in her diet. The key to being your child's nutrition detective is staying open to what the clues could mean and following them through to their logical conclusion.

After six weeks, Tom was an entirely different kid from the one I had met initially, supporting my understanding that his behavior, mood swings, trouble sleeping, and general sickliness all stemmed from his dairy intolerance. In most ways, Tom was cured! He was still a picky eater, but his mother was now excited about improving his diet further. So, back to the clues with an eye toward how to expand his dietary repertoire.

☐ The fact that his twin sister was a good eater suggested that there was not a generally dysfunctional family dynamic around food. Besides, Tom was now more agreeable and started eating better immediately without additional intervention. Reexamining the family situation reminded me that the older brother was also a picky eater.

☐ The specialists had not found any other medical health problem (such as his brother's reflux), so we could cancel out worries about underlying issues. (It is always important to have a doctor or other health care provider check for any other clinical issue that may be affecting your child's health.)

Both his mom and I wanted to round out his diet with more fruits and vegetables and fewer empty-calorie foods such as crackers and cookies. I knew that the more fruits and vegetables he ate, and the more phytonutrients he was provided through these fiber-rich foods, the more calm and well balanced Tom would feel. Based on the clues, I decided we could use behavior modification techniques to introduce new foods.

TAKE CONTROL

The good news is that you don't have to simply accept picky eating as a fact of your child's life. In fact, one of the first things I ask parents to do is take back the control: Children of two, four, six, or eight cannot be left to decide the total composition of their diets. Otherwise, they would generally eat exactly what your picky eater is consuming, such as a bowl of fish-shaped crackers for dinner, as one mother reported. And developmentally, these kinds of bad choices are normal.

What would you eat if you did not know better? In other words, if you couldn't see the connection between eating doughnuts for breakfast and pasta for lunch and feeling tired and cranky and you ate only for taste enjoyment, what would you eat? For me, I confess, it would be ice cream for breakfast and dinner and something warm for lunch. The prefrontal cortex of the brain has the job of tying together your actions with consequences. I know a mostly ice cream diet would make me feel poorly, so I make a conscious choice to refrain. Unfortunately, functional brain studies have shown that the prefrontal cortex does not fully develop until late in the teen years and early twenties. This fact explains much of the obnoxious teenage behavior we observe and also provides the reason why you have to help young children with eating and other decisions until they are capable of making them on their own.

Parents who have no problems telling children to brush their teeth or taking away inappropriate toys suddenly freeze when faced with a child who refuses to eat anything but one brand of frozen pizza for dinner. As one father who had a child-rearing book tucked under his arm when he walked into his appointment observed, "All the experts say you should never make eating a battle. It leads to eating disorders." He, like many other parents, had interpreted this as an admonition not to talk to kids about food or make any dietary demands. I tried to stop myself, but had to ask, "And how is that going for you?"

If you have a picky eater, you have not avoided an eating battle; you are in a continuous one. There may not be active fighting because you have temporarily surrendered, but nobody is winning. Talking about food and telling children they need to eat healthy food does not cause eating disorders any more than educating children about drugs causes addiction. This idea that we need to give children complete control over their food choices might be good for cookie sales, but it is not healthy or developmentally appropriate for them. Some choices, of course; refusing dinner every night unless it is pasta, no way.

NUTRITION DETECTIVE
PRINCIPLE #3

With picky eaters, take small, consistent steps.

Judging by the six- to twelve-month waiting lists at hospital-based programs for picky eaters, I would classify picky eating in this generation as an epidemic. Most parents are unsuccessful with eating issues because the steps they are taking are too big and overwhelm the picky eater, and they are not prepared for how long it can take to change habits. When I was an undergraduate, we were taught that picky eating was caused by parents indulging kids' natural tendency to restrict their food choices. Believe it or not, this viewpoint prevails in the medical world even today. Blaming the parents grossly oversimplifies a complicated issue and is not making the problem go away. Small, consistent steps made by both parents and kids will lead to success.

Now don't panic; I'm not suggesting an endless food fight or a siege in which the child is left to starve unless she eats the spiced lentils. Rather, I'm going to share with you a three-step plan that can soothe even the pickiest eater. It is the middle way. No fighting, no surrendering. Think of this approach as a peace plan for the dinner table that works. I call this plan the E.A.T. program—more on it in chapter 4. Because Tom was now more emotionally stable, I suggested that with his mom's help, he begin to add some new foods to his diet, one food, one bite at a time.

Keep in mind, it's always much easier to work on making changes with kids when they are not physically uncomfortable. The main reason Tom was calmer and easier to work with was that, having removed from his diet the dairy he was unable to digest, he was no longer in pain. If only he could have just told his parents that he did not feel well before! But like most kids, Tom didn't know how to articulate how bad he was feeling—mostly because he had no basis of comparison. In hindsight, his behavior and body were screaming what his mouth could not say. We just had to follow the clues.

Of course, there are a hundred reasons why kids feel and act bad. But most kids, depending on their age and the nature of the problem, have difficulty pinpointing an area of discomfort or explaining what feels so bad. The universal language for children is their behavior. Children are giving you clues and trying to tell you something through their behavior; they are not bad. They are more like puppies that cannot articulate their discomfort any other way.

There are many types of discomfort, including psychological discomfort. Children can be sad, anxious, or traumatized and behave badly in response, just like the rest of us. Sometimes they are overindulged, or perhaps they have an inflexible nature. Some of these behaviors are pathological, but many involve difficult but normal variations in human conduct. The problem is when psychological labels become the fallback position because biological causes are believed to have been ruled out—another case of not knowing what we do not know. Psychological diagnoses can become a confusing wild card in unraveling children's issues because they certainly exist, but in my opinion are used too often.

Psychological issues must be acknowledged and given their due, but this book focuses mostly on how biological and nutritional imbalances can cause psychological and behavioral issues, with the clear understanding that the river flows both ways.

Is Your Child a Picky Eater?

The way I see it, if your child restricts her food choices and is not getting a balanced diet that includes vegetables, fruits, and whole grains, and if at the same time she relies on sugary and starchy foods, then you may have a picky eater who needs to change her habits. Find out by answering the following questions:

☐ Does your child lack vitality?

☐ Does your child look sickly or unhealthy?

☐ Is your child moody or overly sensitive?

☐ Does your child eat a mostly "white" diet—bread, pasta, crackers, white cheese?

☐ Do you find yourself wondering in the morning if this will be a "good" or "bad" day?

☐ Does your child complain that many foods taste or smell funny?

☐ Is your child unable to eat foods or dishes that are mixed, such as meat loaf, or salad with various vegetables included?

☐ Are mealtimes stressful because of food negotiating/refusal?

☐ Do you have to prepare a separate dinner for your child most nights?

If you answered yes to two or more of these questions, you likely have a picky eater.

What to Do

1. If you think your child is suffering from an irritant, consider these symptoms: pale, pasty-looking complexion; skin anomalies (eczema, hives, dermatitis, rashes); bowel issues, especially constipation, or frequent diarrhea (a sign of gluten intolerance); sick all the time; craving beyond reason dairy or wheat-based products.

2. Next, consult a health care professional such as a nutritionist, GI specialist, or allergist to discuss testing possibilities or questions that need answering. The best test, however, is simple: eliminating the food you suspect. That way you can see your child's individual response.

3. Try a simple elimination diet for four to six weeks. Dairy is the most common food irritant, followed by sugar and gluten and wheat-based foods.

4. If you eliminate dairy, replace the calcium with 900–1,000 milligrams of calcium supplement, split into two doses. Don't substitute soy milk for dairy, because soy has a similar chemical structure to milk, so half of kids with dairy issues have the same response to soy. The soy/dairy relationship is discussed further in chapter 5.

5. Then try the E.A.T. program discussed in the next chapter, along with a multivitamin that includes 15 milligrams of zinc if the child is three or older.

CHAPTER 4

The E.A.T. Program: What It Is and How It Works

I MET MARCO WHEN HE WAS ALMOST ELEVEN. He was of normal weight, but ate only three foods (pasta, yogurt, and bagels) and had begun to feel awkward socially because of his very limited palate. His parents had visited several psychologists and doctors about the problem, to no avail. Whether or not Marco would attend an event had more to do with the food being served than the activity itself—he was nervous that someone would ask him to try something. If he was invited to a party, he had to check ahead to make sure they'd be serving a food that he'd eat. This is not as rare a situation as you might think.

Marco explained very honestly that he wanted to eat more foods and try new things, but couldn't get himself to do it. Just talking about peanut butter brought tears to his eyes! His parents wanted to help because they worried that in the teenage years his eating habits would become an even bigger social liability. "If only pizza was one of the three foods he ate," they lamented. His parents admitted they had finally just thrown up their hands in defeat, figuring he would eventually grow up and perhaps spontaneously decide to try new foods then.

In my assessment, I picked out two clues to follow: one, Marco was literally disgusted by many foods; and two, although he had become very anxious about even *thinking* about trying a new food, he seemed to want to change this attitude. Because so many foods disgusted him, clue number one made me think about zinc. Children with a deficiency of the mineral zinc can become almost repelled by the tastes or smells of many foods. Marco's "white" diet did not contain zinc (and many other minerals); people with low levels of zinc can lose their senses of smell and taste or have those senses altered, causing them to experience normal foods in unpleasant or unusual ways. So the first thing I did was put Marco on a multivitamin with zinc to improve his sense of taste and smell. (See page 112 for more information on testing of zinc levels.) Because of his poor diet, his mother had been giving him a chewable kids' multivitamin for years, but it had only 2 milligrams of zinc. The supplement I suggested provided a better spectrum of minerals and, most important, 15 milligrams of zinc.

In response to clue number two, I had him take a specially formulated fish oil to address anxiety. Many studies have demonstrated the positive effect of one of the fats in fish oil (called EPA) on anxiety, mood, and behavior. Marco's limited diet was completely devoid of basic essential fats, including the omega-3 fats found in fish and seaweed. Fats are structural nutrients that affect the way the brain operates and are calming. If we could not help Marco reduce his emotional stress around eating, we were not going to be successful at introducing new foods. You will read the details of how omega-3 fatty acids affect anxiety in chapter 13.

To support him further, we put together the "one food, one bite" plan for introducing new foods. I asked him, "Do you think it would be possible to try just one bite of the same food every day for a few weeks?" This is a good technique for getting extremely picky eaters to change their habits over time. Generally, I let adolescents choose the new food or try to choose

Children with a deficiency of the mineral zinc can become almost repelled by the tastes or smells of many foods.

a food similar to something they already eat. Younger kids need more direction and ideas. Try to limit your food suggestions to two so the child is not overwhelmed by too many choices.

The foods Marco wanted to learn to eat, such as pizza and hamburgers, were too intimidating to start with, so I suggested radishes. This is an unusual first trial food, but radishes are mostly white and have a strong flavor, and Marco had no emotional history or thoughts about them. Many other therapists had tried and failed with more traditional bland foods such as applesauce and adding cheese to his pasta. I figured the radishes were worth a try.

I warned Marco that he would probably gag the first several days and that this was normal. He was shaky but reluctantly agreed to stick with only one bite of a slice of radish for two weeks. And he did! Marco did indeed gag and shake every day during the first week when he put the bite of food into his mouth. The key to his success was based on both his surviving the gagging and his parents remaining serene, even when his anxiety increased. I told his parents they had to stay absolutely calm and tell him he could do it even though he was struggling like crazy. Repeating the small successes (one bite) gradually helped him develop a healthy acclimation to eating new foods. Slowly, through the first two weeks, he grew accustomed to both the idea of trying a new food and the experience of eating a new food. He did not like gagging, but rather than seeing it as a signal to stop immediately, he saw it as something he could overcome. By the end of the month, he rarely retched when trying new foods. I often remind parents that acclimation will happen, but that it can take time and effort.

Marco and his parents stuck with the program, not stopping with one successful food, but using the positive experience to continue introducing new foods. It turned out that Marco had spent a lot of time "watching food," and when it came time to try the next few new foods, he chose them. Marco ended up liking (and eating) duck, hamburgers, and mustard! He did not like radishes but overall preferred strong flavors—showing that not all kids prefer sweet foods. With his preferences in mind, we looked for other foods to awaken his taste buds.

THE E.A.T. PROGRAM

Improving the diet of a picky eater—or any child lacking in nutrients—is difficult but necessary and possible. With both Tom and Marco, I followed the clues that their behavior and diet were suggesting, eliminated irritants when necessary, waited for or helped the boys to calm down and feel better enough, and then began adding foods and other supplements to further improve their nutritional status and all-around health. My basic strategy, and one that I have successfully used with hundreds of picky eaters, is designated by the acronym E.A.T. Follow it, and before you know it you will have a child who . . . eats!

E—Eliminate any irritants that may be causing a bad reaction.

A—Add one food at a time.

T—Try one bite of this food each night for two weeks.

The basis of this program is that kids need time to get used to foods that are unfamiliar or otherwise distasteful. Food preferences develop through a process of acclimation. People get used to what they have been exposed to and tend to prefer the known. Thus, Irish people tend to like potatoes, Chinese people eat rice rather than bread with meals, people growing up in the South eat turnips, and so on. The observation is not an attempt to defend cultural stereotypes but an acknowledgment that people tend to like what they know.

You can't expect any child to embrace a food at first glance, never mind first bite. In Mexico, mothers put hot sauce on babies' lips at nine months old. Of course the babies often scowl, but the mothers persevere, because eating food spiced with hot peppers is part of their cultural diet and children need to get used to it. In the United States, we shy away from this kind of training. If Mikey doesn't like the first taste of peas, we announce that Mikey does not like peas and tend not to try them again, so Mikey never has a chance to actually grow accustomed to peas. He becomes a pea-avoiding adolescent (or a broccoli-hating president). Should ten-month-old children really make that decision? They often do in Western cultures, and we have an epidemic of picky eaters in this generation to prove it.

Resisting the urge to respond immediately to a child's initial dislike of a food takes a lot of patience on the part of parents and caregivers. And although the E.A.T program works, it does require you to stay calm, cool, and collected and to persevere. Don't stop after one success or failure—keep going!

The E.A.T. program works like this:

1. You **Eliminate** any irritant, or in some cases unhealthy food, from your child's diet.

2. You explain to your child that for the next two weeks, he is going to **Add** one new food. (You help your child decide on this food, making it somewhat similar in texture, color, or taste to a food he already enjoys.)

3. You then explain that all you are asking for him to do is **Try** one bite of the new food. He will be trying one bite of the same new food every day for two weeks.

One mother brought her seven-year-old daughter, Claudia, to see me because she and her husband were heartsick with worry about Claudia's pickiness around food. Like many children, Claudia ate everything until she was two, at which point her diet was reduced to your typical kids' menu: pancakes, cookies, sugared cereal, chicken nuggets, mac-and-cheese, pizza. No fruit. No vegetables. No fish. No whole grains, legumes, or mixed dishes. She was extremely sensitive to smells, often constipated, and had trouble going to sleep. As an only child, Claudia had all her parents' attention; she became hysterical when asked to try a new food, and her parents backed off immediately.

We all know that food and eating provides one of the first and most stubborn battlegrounds for kids, which makes sense, developmentally. At two years old, most kids notice that when they do something, they get a reaction. If they put a sneaker in the toilet, it makes a fun sound trying to go down the pipe. Isn't that interesting? They begin to wonder what else they control, because clearly there is some control to be had. This is a normal part of development.

Very frustrating for toddlers, most events seem to be under the control of the big people. The giants force them into car seats, shove them into strollers, and put them to bed when they don't want to go, and there is not a darn thing they can do about it. Screaming does not seem to help very much. But, what is this? Close my mouth and the food goes away? Finally, something a two-year-old can control. This is why so many kids are such good eaters until age two.

Unlike Tom, whom we met earlier, Claudia was not moody or difficult, nor was she sick often (though she was often constipated). In fact, she was a sweet little darling beloved by both friends and teachers. However, her mother began to panic when she started getting reports from school about her deteriorating attention span. As the demands increased, Claudia was not able to follow directions and seemed to be increasingly in her own world.

In this case, the first clue I followed was how easily upset Claudia's parents became: They panicked right alongside their daughter when she struggled with eating. I figured that their reaction was not helping anyone. We reviewed the E.A.T. program, and I gave Claudia's parents their marching orders: Claudia could learn to eat new foods, but they would have to be able to tolerate her initial distress when trying a new food. Under no circumstance were they to stop trying a new food just because Claudia found it difficult.

After three visits, over three months, Claudia had not only begun to eat the "one bite" but had discovered some healthy foods she liked. The reports stopped coming home from school, and as her diet continued to improve, she began to listen better and follow directions better, and overall seemed more alert and resilient.

How did Claudia improve so quickly on the E.A.T. program? She did not have irritants in her diet per se, but she was consuming a lot of empty calories. It is always easier to *eliminate* junk than to *add* healthy foods. Therefore, for the first step—Eliminate—I suggested removing the worst of the empty-calorie junk foods from her diet because they were adding no nutritional value, but were taking up stomach space. We eliminated sugary breakfast foods and desserts.

At the second step—Add—we added eggs and then carrots (one at a time). We asked her whether she would rather practice eating eggs or chicken for the first food. She was too upset to answer, so her father chose eggs and told her she could pick the second practice food. Once the one bite of egg was taken every day for two weeks, he offered her a choice of two vegetables (carrots or lettuce). She picked carrots.

For the third step—Try—her parents told her she needed to try just one bite of the practice food. She tried the bite, but only after a couple of days of howling and copious tears. Her parents did not jump to her rescue as she expected but stayed strangely calm and encouraged her to keep going. With nothing else to do, Claudia began to try the "icky" new food.

When she stopped relying on an empty-calorie kid diet made up of low-fiber white foods, which was keeping her constipated, which in turn kept her from sleeping soundly, her system regulated within a couple of weeks.

Sound simple? It is. Here's why.

How many times has a parent lamented, "I just want him to eat *something*" to justify a diet of junk food meals, cookies, and ice cream? Although it takes time to retrain your child's brain (the main obstacle to his trying and enjoying a variety of foods), it is easy to take away the worst of the empty calories. If a child will eat only peanut butter and jelly sandwiches and desserts, then eliminate desserts. Better to eat peanut butter and jelly three times a day than to have only one real meal and the rest of the diet be filler nonfoods, like crackers and cookies.

This single step can improve the diet 100 percent. Foods that contain calories but are limited in nutrients can be dangerous when a child is a picky eater. Nature is not wasteful. It expects all of your food to contain some of what you need. A peanut butter sandwich has some of the nutrients you need for the day, but if the rest of the diet provides

WHEN TRYING NEW FOODS, GO FOR SOMETHING FAMILIAR

Some experts call this food chaining. The principle is that the new food should have some characteristics of a food already eaten. If a child eats only mushy foods, you would not pick a crunchy carrot as a trial item. Pick something with a similar color and texture or taste and color. Here are some examples:

- If your child loves french fries, try sweet-potato fries.

- If she likes the crunchiness of chips, try baked or freeze-dried vegetables.

- If he likes crackers, try multigrain crackers.

- If he likes soft mac-and-cheese, try squash soup, which is creamy in texture.

almost no nutrients, you have a situation where a child is trying to grow and learn on perhaps 25 or 30 percent of the nutrients normally required.

Sugar, in particular, has been proven to be as addicting as heroin in some people (and certainly in rats). If cookies and ice cream were nutritionally complete, there would be no such thing as picky eaters, because most of them love sweets. Those who don't have a sweet tooth tend to prefer white, starchy food such as pasta and bread. Interestingly, in more than twenty-five years I have only once had a parent express concern about her child because he wanted spinach every day. I assured the anxious parent that this choice was not a problem. If your child refuses chips but insists on broccoli or green beans, give this book to someone else (or at least skip this chapter)!

If you cut out the junk and your child gets bored eating pizza three times a day, then that is an opportunity to introduce a new food.

You have to keep introducing new items to your picky eater, trusting that you will find one he likes, and you will. Most parents have "tried" to the point of bitter frustration with no real progress. Successful food trials require you to do the following:

- Give the child a choice of two foods to try so he still has some control over eating. If he refuses to choose, tell him you will pick the first one and he can pick the second. Keep choosing for him until he joins in.

- Choose a food with some familiar characteristics and try it at one meal or snack time for two weeks.

- Introduce each food one by one.

- Be consistent, letting your child acclimate to the one food for ten to fourteen days.

- If your child tolerates that food, keep it as a standard offering. If he doesn't tolerate it, after two weeks, choose another food and discontinue the first.

- Provide incentives: Let your child know that when he is finished with his one bite, he will be able to watch a favorite program, play outside, or enjoy some other reward, depending on his desire. When trying to figure out the incentive that will work best for your child, ask yourself, Why should my child change her behavior? If everything stays the same and nothing happens if she does not cooperate, why should she? The best consequences are logical and follow naturally: "When you finish with this, we can do that."

And remember, it's okay to let your child struggle with the job of taking one bite. Above all, remain calm and keep introducing new foods.

TIPS FOR MAKING E.A.T. WORK

You have to be consistent, which means one food at a time over a period of two weeks. Picky eaters don't like food surprises. Knowing they will be dealing with the same new food for two weeks helps them calm down because they are forewarned. They need to be eased into a new experience. Anxiety about the new is reduced with frequent repetition. Tell your child that she will be making one "try" bite of whatever food you choose. Keep it positive. Provide the food every day for at least

When Picky Eating Means Something More Serious

Symptoms that suggest there are underlying problems with the ability to eat that need to be addressed, especially before starting the E.A.T. program, include the following:

- excessive drooling

- child has never progressed past baby food textures: mostly eats mushy foods

- bad or acidy breath

- a diagnosis of sensory processing disorder, autism, or excessive sensory reactions to many situations beyond eating

- child takes much longer to eat than seems normal

- child gags or vomits frequently

- child pockets food in the cheeks

- child complains frequently of stomachaches

- child refuses to touch most foods or sit at a table containing new foods

If your child exhibits any of these symptoms, I recommend that you seek a health care professional's advice before attempting new foods. If your child does not have any of these symptoms but you are still uncertain, get help.

ten to fourteen days. After a few weeks, the child will be familiar with the food and will like it or not. Even if children tolerate the new item, they may not request a large serving. Still, the new food is now in the child's diet. One child I worked with was as stubborn as they come. At eight years old, Grace ate only chicken nuggets, pasta with butter, and occasionally, pizza. The mother was resigned to the situation, but once she observed that her daughter was putting on weight, she decided to get help. We went through a typical line of questioning to follow the clues, and it became clear that much like Claudia, Grace was lacking in both essential fatty acids and zinc.

In six weeks of using the E.A.T. program, Grace tried and successfully added three new foods: romaine lettuce, fish sticks, and apples. At my suggestion, her mother also gave her fish oil supplements and a multivitamin with zinc. As Grace recently said to me, she doesn't *love* the fish sticks she tried, but she now eats them without a fuss. "They're not my favorite, but I like them enough" was the comment. You don't eat your favorite foods every night, right?

With Grace, as with most children, it was acclimation and insistence that worked. It also helped that her mom was consistent and calm, and set up clear consequences. Consequences should not be presented as a reward or a punishment; they are the next thing that happens, which is being controlled and articulated by the parent. In the best scenario there is a sequence that follows logically, such as, "When you are done eating your bite of squash, then we can go outside and play." This is quite different than saying, "If you don't eat that squash, there will be no playing outside tonight." The setup changes how you and the result are perceived by the child. To avoid control issues with food, you should be neither a punisher nor a rewarder. Allow the natural consequences of the child's choices (which are being orchestrated by you) to be the incentive. The choice to eat the squash means there will be time to play outside, while procrastinating and crying means there will be no time left for play. If you present the situation with a reward or punishment at the end, you position yourself as an adversary rather than a supporter.

Most picky eaters will not readily attempt new foods unless there is a good reason to do so. Thus consequences become the tipping factor. What happens when the little one does not cooperate? If when she pitches a screaming fit you succumb and remove the food and give her something else, she learns that pitching a fit clearly works!

I've said it before, and I'll say it again—the most important thing is for parents to stay *calm* as their child goes through the sensory distress of trying a new food. Yes, your child might cry a little bit—it's okay. Instead of feeding into her panic or nervousness by becoming nervous yourself, be reassuring. Yes, the texture of the tomato feels different; yes, the red pepper has a slightly spicy smell. Refer to the last time your child tried something different and remind her she can be successful.

However, explanations are not a substitute for a calm presence and logical consequences. Or as they say in the East, talk does not cook the rice. Most children need a reason to make a change, and the best reason is a consequence. One could argue that most people will not take on difficult tasks without a consequence. How many of us would bother doing the very hard thing of writing a check for our taxes if there was not a consequence for failure to pay? The parent has to provide a reason for the child to tackle the hard process of eating new foods. If pleasing Mom were enough of an incentive, the child would not be a fussy eater. The best consequence, because it follows naturally, is not starting the next desired activity until the child is ready. *Ready* is defined by the parent as the child finishing the one bite of the new food.

The evening's activities need to be kept on hold until the child's job (i.e., taking the one bite) is done. Psychologists call this technique when/then. "When you are finished with your dinner, then you can turn on the computer." This is preferable to "If you would only eat your stupid green beans, we could go to the park."

Again, it's okay to let your child struggle as he tries to take the one bite. Don't run in to cajole, rescue, distract, or push. Life should not revolve around a child refusing to eat. Pay your bills. Call your sister. And occasionally, remind your child that you are ready to turn on the TV (or whatever the next activity is) when he is finished.

When it comes to food, we forget the lessons we know from experience: We are able to suffer through a child's temper tantrum. After all, we wouldn't hesitate to stick to our guns if our child threw a fit that endangered his safety. For many of us food represents love, so making demands about it is uncomfortable, and parents have a hard time calming themselves down when a child refuses to eat. Instead, parents mistakenly believe that having any household rules about food will cause an eating disorder.

The worst thing that will happen if you insist that your child take a bite is that the child will throw up. And if that's the case, then resort to what I call "the Meryl Streep school of acting." Pretend nothing alarming has occurred, put on a straight face, and say, "Oh, dear, the food fell out. We'll just have to try this again tomorrow." Your child needs to know that throwing up is not what she has to do to stop the program. However, if your child continues to throw up several days in a row or develops escalating behavioral problems, you must have a professional eating evaluation. (See "When Picky Eating Means Something More Serious" on page 58 for further information.) Some children literally do not have the physical skills for easy chewing and swallowing, and the introduction of new foods can cause panic attacks. If at any point you feel the situation is getting out of hand, contact a speech therapist, occupational therapist, or other professional with training in eating, chewing, and sensory issues. She will watch your child eat and determine if there are underlying problems that should be addressed before using a structured behavioral approach. I have several therapists I refer patients to for this purpose, and it is surprising how often kids have a developmental quirk that makes the process of eating difficult.

Borrowing from the television psychotherapist Dr. Phil, here is a sample script for walking through consequences. The script begins after a food has been decided upon and the child is refusing to eat it.

Mother: As soon as you are finished eating your one bite of carrot, I will read you another chapter in your dragon book.

Child: I don't want to eat a carrot tonight. It has a spot on it. I will eat another carrot tomorrow.

Mother: I see you are not ready to read yet because you haven't finished your bite. I hope you finish soon so we do not run out of time to read before bed. Let me know when you are ready. I will be washing dishes over here.

Child (after glaring at the carrot and kicking the table leg for ten minutes): I hate carrots, and I don't care about reading my stupid dragon book.

Mother: That is too bad because I wanted to know what happens next, but if you do not finish in time for reading tonight, we can always try again tomorrow.

Child (now crying): It is too hard, and I will never finish in time. WAAAAAAAAA!

Mother continues to wash dishes without looking up.

Child: WAAAAAA?

Mother: Are you finished yet?

Child makes a face but takes a tiny bite.

Mother: Good job. Let's go read.

Once children see that the parent is not reacting and resistance is futile, they usually calm down and get the job done, unless there are other underlying problems. For the most part, by the third new food trial the habit of trying a new food is getting established and there is less resistance, especially if the parents have been consistent about having them take one bite. If the child becomes increasingly hysterical no matter how

EVERY CHILD SHOULD TAKE A MULTIVITAMIN

For good measure and optimal health, all kids should take a multivitamin on a daily basis at best, or at least two or three times a week. But not all kids' multis contain enough of the minerals and vitamins you are looking for. Most ingredients in a child's multivitamin are measured as a percentage of a mysterious standard called the Daily Value (DV). The DVs are general recommendations for what constitutes a healthy diet that are vague, extremely general ballpark estimates of what is usually enough to prevent deficiency, and do not take into account any individual needs.

When you are choosing a good multivitamin, consider these qualities:

- Make sure it contains vitamin C (go for 100 milligrams if you can find it)

- Vitamin E (recommended amount)

- Vitamin A levels previously considered desirable (about 5,000 IUs) are now thought to be too much for younger children, although many multis still contain high levels. Look for 2,500 IUs or less.

- Be sure the multi you choose contains the full set of B-vitamins— B1, B2, niacinamide, B5, B6, folic acid, and B12. (Know that gummy vitamins tend to be missing B-vitamins.)

calm you are, refuses to even touch the food, or screams for more than fifteen minutes, get professional help.

SUPPLEMENTS TO SUPPORT A PICKY EATER

Nutritional supplements can close the gap between what a child is willing to eat and what she needs for brain development. Picky eating can be a vicious cycle if a child becomes significantly malnourished. Malnutrition itself can lead to picky eating and more malnutrition. In zinc deficiency, for example, taste becomes altered so that food tastes bland or smells "off." The child then restricts the diet further, leading to more severe nutritional imbalances. (See chapter 7 for more about zinc and appetite.) Low levels of other nutrients can also negatively affect the desire to eat. Most picky eaters, who are three or older, even if they

- Calcium is almost never present in significant amounts in children's multis; you need to supplement so your child gets at least 800–1,000 milligrams of total calcium between his diet and the supplement. Extra calcium is mostly a concern for children on dairy-free diets or those who do not like milk products.

- Most multis for kids are weak in minerals. Try to find one that includes zinc, selenium, magnesium, and chromium.

- Most children's multis contain 200–400 IUs of vitamin D even though most health care professionals now believe 800–1,000 IUs is a better goal. You may need to add extra, which is available in drops.

- If your child is gluten-intolerant or has other food reactions, make sure the multi doesn't contain trace amounts of flour, corn, dairy, and other potentially allergic substances. Many of the better companies help by saying "Does not contain [gluten, dairy, soy, etc.]" clearly on the label.

When possible, avoid artificial colors and flavors and the gummy variety of children's multi. Although the artificial flavors cover the vitamin-y taste, they can be irritating or cause allergic reactions in young children. (For more complete information about my recommendations on kids' multivitamins, see page 297.)

NUTRITION DETECTIVE
PRINCIPLE #4

Our children watch our every move.

Why? Because they are using our cues to help them decide on the proper reaction. Picky eaters are typically highly sensitive creatures who are wired to piggyback off their parents' reactions. They rely on their parents to help self-regulate. The less upset you seem, and the less angry and frustrated you become, the calmer your child will be. This principle applies not only to dealing with the picky eater but also to managing any kind of child whose diet you seek to change.

are not being bothered by an irritant, should take a multivitamin/mineral that has more than 100 percent of the Daily Value for all the B-vitamins and at least 15 milligrams of zinc. The Daily Value is the bare minimum standard set to avoid deficiency syndromes in "most" people and should not be used as a measure of optimal intake. Many of the popular gummy vitamins are poor choices because they do not contain a full spectrum of B-vitamins. Be sure the supplement contains vitamins B1, B2, B5, B6, and B12, as well as folic acid and niacinamide.

Trying foods with familiar qualities, consistent exposure, and immediate consequences is the key to avoiding food fights. Combined with eliminating any irritating foods (or ones that are empty of good nutrition, such as baked snack foods and sweets), the E.A.T. program can turn around the fussiest eater within weeks!

When the Body Behaves Badly

CHAPTER 5

The Toddler Who Could Not Stop Spitting Up

W HEN I FIRST STARTED PRACTICING more than twenty-five years ago, babies who spit up were rarely treated medically. The thinking was that most babies spit up and that it was normal. If mothers complained to their pediatricians or expressed worry that their babies weren't taking in enough nutrition, they were told simply that their babies would outgrow the behavior. In other words, it was just a phase. Today there is a trend to diagnose any kind of spitting up as reflux (properly called gastroesophageal reflux disease, or GERD) and to treat it medically.

By definition, it is GERD only if there is pain and irritation in the nose and mouth along with other symptoms such as chronic coughing or feeding problems. But the strict definition of GERD is rarely applied to a screeching infant, because that would require an endoscopy for confirmation. An endoscopy involves threading a small camera down the little one's throat after knocking her out. Doctors do not like to do this before age one, and you can imagine how popular such a suggestion would be among new parents. Instead, whether a baby is screaming because the act of throwing up is frightening or she is uncomfortable because the regurgitated lunch is burning her throat, she is treated for reflux. One study followed forty-four spitting-up infants. Forty-two of the infants were already on medicine when the study started, but only eight actually had GERD when fully tested. In other words, only 20 percent of the babies treated for reflux actually had reflux.

WHY IS REFLUX SO COMMON?

How prevalent is reflux in babies? Neither the Centers for Disease Control and Prevention nor the National Center for Health Statistics have quotable data. I know this because I called them when I could not find anything reliable. Nonetheless, there is no shortage

---

A REFLUX PRIMER

The stomach is like a drawstring bag. The top or drawstring part is called the lower esophageal sphincter (LES). A sphincter is a muscular structure that operates like a door in body passages or at orifices. The most well-known body sphincter is the anus. The lesser-known LES is the door between the esophagus (the food pipe leading to the tummy) and the stomach. It is the band of muscles that opens and closes when a person swallows. In GERD, the LES is not able to create the necessary seal, so it leaks. The leak allows the acidy contents of the stomach to seep up into the esophagus, which is not coated to protect against acid. The esophagus uses its layer of muscle to move food from the mouth to the stomach, pushing food and saliva down into the stomach. The stomach normally continues this process by pushing food farther along the digestive tract into the small intestine. Because the stomach has stretched like a balloon to accommodate the food, pressure develops. If there is too much pressure in the stomach, the LES cannot keep the food in the stomach, and up it comes. Sometimes, pressure can occur as a result of an inflammation of the gut lining—an irritated gut lining works to rid itself of the food nuisance.

How high can the pressure be? High enough to project stomach contents into the sinuses. In rare cases specks of lunch can end up in the lungs, leading to dangerous complications such as pneumonia. In babies, where the distance between the tummy and mouth is tiny and muscles are underdeveloped, the food flies out easily.

of figures bandied about online. The Children's Digestive Health and Nutrition Foundation claims more than 50 percent of babies spit up regularly in the first months of life. Another source claims that 20 percent of the eight million babies born every year suffer from reflux. (This source's website counted a manufacturer of reflux medicine among its sponsors.)

Some doctors make the distinction between so-called normal spitting up and reflux based on whether or not the child is happy (and spitting up) or distressed (and spitting up). The happy spitter-uppers are not medicated if they are gaining weight properly and are comfortable. They are expected to outgrow the condition.

And outgrow it they do. The reliable statistics for outgrowing reveal that 80 percent of children stop having reflux symptoms by age one and 95 percent of reflux resolves by age two without doing anything at all.

Physiological problems can cause reflux. Excessive fat around the waist, for example, squishes the stomach and puts more pressure on the LES, increasing the chances of leakage. This is the most common reason for reflux in adults, and sadly, is becoming more of a problem for children as more of them become obese. In children, the physiological problems are more often caused by low muscle tone or birth defects. In some birth defects the spine is crooked, compressing the stomach into a shape that increases pressure on the LES. When the muscles around the stomach are underdeveloped or do not have enough tone, they do not hold the soft stomach in place, putting more pressure on the sphincter.

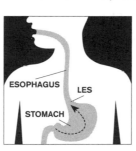

Reflux occurs when food mixed with acid backs up from the stomach, past the lower esophageal sphincter (LES) and into the esophagus.

When the muscle tone is low enough, the child can literally be slumped over, again stressing the LES. Low muscle tone can be a factor in many genetic conditions such as Down syndrome, and birth defects such as cerebral palsy. There are also rare instances when some part of the digestive system did not form correctly in utero, causing problems that only surgery can correct.

But the key thing to keep in mind is that medications are being prescribed for GERD in infants when they are simply spitting up.

69

Those numbers stand as testament to the fact that the doctors of yore were mostly right—spitting up is just a phase. Mostly. What complicates matters today is the stubborn trend of over-medicalizing the treatment of spitting up. Today's moms are more medically aware thanks to rampant drug advertising and popular medical TV programs such as *The Doctors* or *Grey's Anatomy*. They have not only heard of reflux, but know the names of the medicines used to treat it. As soon as that first dollop of spit-up lands on their shoulder, some of these moms run to their pediatricians, prediagnosing their children with reflux and asking for the medicine. Even if the pediatrician knows better, she may still offer the baby medicine because the parents request it, with the caveat that if he does not get better, a specialist should be consulted. One of the potential dangers or triggers for confusion, however, comes if the child's symptoms go away; then mother and doctor often jump to the conclusion that the child was indeed suffering from reflux.

Unfortunately, just because a child's symptoms are temporarily mitigated by reflux medicine, that does not mean he actually has reflux or that the underlying issue is being addressed. Thus a large number of infants end up on reflux medicine and sometimes, like Molly, whom we'll meet below, cannot seem to get off it.

MOLLY'S MEDICINE

Babies who are put on medicine to treat reflux often end up in my office when they're around two or three years of age. Molly was one of these youngsters. An adorable blonde two-year-old, Molly had been on her reflux medicine since she was four months old because of excessive crying, spitting up, and poor weight gain. The medicine barely reduced her symptoms, but her mom and dad were afraid to take her off it because whenever they tried, Molly became even more miserable. They brought her in because even at the highest dose of medication the specialist prescribed, she was still cranky and uncomfortable much of the time, and always constipated. They were also worried that Molly had never gained

How Reflux Drugs Work

There are two main types of medicines used for reflux: acid suppressants and antisecretory agents. You probably know about acid suppressants, aka antacids, which can be purchased in little Lifesaver-like rolls at any drugstore. They soak up acid after the fact and are very popular with people who want to be able to eat whatever or as much as they want. When the inevitable heartburn follows, the sufferer simply pops a few antacids. Doctors rarely use them to treat reflux anymore. They prefer to use stronger medicines that do not buffer acid already in the stomach but stop its production.

Antisecretory agents act by stopping the release of acid, so the problem stops before it starts. There are two types of antisecretory agents: histamine-2 receptor antagonists (H2 blockers) such as famotidine (Pepcid), cimetidine (Tagamet), rantidine (Zantac), and nizatidine (Axid), and proton pump inhibitors (PPIs) such as omeprazole (Prilosec) and lansoprazole (Prevacid). H2 blockers are the weaker acid-secretion blockers and are usually prescribed first. PPIs are very strong and stop the mechanism that pumps acid into the stomach.

Long-term use of these drugs causes nutritional deficiencies, because stomach acid is needed to properly absorb protein, calcium, zinc, vitamin B12, and other nutrients. They can also cause neurological side effects such as headaches and the sensation of a lump in the throat. There is even a class action suit regarding one particular drug known to cause a serious movement disorder. Better to consider medicine as a short-term palliative solution while you continue to look for the cause of the reflux.

weight properly or steadily (at twenty-four months, she weighed only eighteen pounds) and was uninterested in eating. She was so underweight that her parents believed she was slowly starving. Because Molly had no interest in eating and was eating less and less, her pediatrician had put her on a high-calorie milk-based drink several months before to maintain her caloric intake.

Her pediatrician had sent Molly to a gastrointestinal (GI) specialist, who supervised a plan to reduce the medication because she was taking so much with so little benefit. She cried and fussed worse than ever. The specialist finally insisted on an endoscopy, which found severe irritation in her esophagus, despite aggressive medicating.

THE SCOOP ON SCOPES

An endoscopic procedure is a way for doctors to peek inside the body rather than continue to guess about the source of the problem based on a patient's reported complaints. For simple gastrointestinal procedures, a thin, flexible instrument is inserted into a natural opening. If that natural opening is the mouth, the specialist is examining the esophagus, stomach, and duodenum (known as an upper GI endoscopy). If it is the rectum, it is a colonoscopy. Lung specialists use the nose for their internal journey and prefer a special fiber-optic bronchoscope to check out the windpipe (trachea) and the bronchi. Little miniature garden tool–like attachments at the end of the scopes can collect tissue samples, snip off polyps, or remove pennies and other foreign items that do not belong there.

Just thinking about a doctor holding a tube, let alone inserting it, makes many people break out in a cold sweat, so some level of sedation is necessary to relax the patient. In addition, the section of the GI tract one wishes to study must be cleared of debris. For an upper-GI endoscopy, fasting after midnight usually does the trick. A colonoscopy requires a more stringent cleaning using benignly named laxatives, such as GoLYTELY. Nobody would use a product called Lots of Diarrhea, but most parents quickly figure out that these cleverly named laxatives are very strong and worry about using them with young children. Sedation and colon preparation usually concern parents more than the procedure itself, which has limited risks when performed by a competent physician.

The doctor tried several new reflux medicines with no improvement. In addition, Molly had already been seeing a feeding therapist to address some of the behavioral issues that were developing around eating, including shaking her head when her mom tried to feed her. Yes, Molly's mother was still mostly hand-feeding her, because Molly was trying to wander away from the table at dinnertime, and in general was seemingly not hungry or interested in food.

Unable to help the girl medically, nutrition intervention seemed the next logical step, so the gastroenterologist sent the parents to me.

When I read the GI specialist's report on Molly, I discovered that Molly's esophagus was lined with white blood cells. The presence of white blood cells meant that her body was responding to some kind of infection, injury, and/or allergy. The doctor's diagnosis of GERD was based on her presumption that the leakage was the main problem, but I was not so sure. If just stopping the backup was the full issue, the medicine should have worked. The bigger question was why Molly's stomach continued to be irritated. Many diagnoses, such as reflux, are more accurately descriptions of the symptoms rather than an explanation of the root cause of a problem.

I remember one doctor friend quipping, "The name is the game. That is the way we were taught." In other words, the main concern in medical practice is to identify the correct diagnosis, because by definition it should lead to the correct treatment. However, if the diagnosis does not tell you why something is happening, the description of the symptoms can lead to palliative measures, but not corrective treatment. Getting rid of pain is good for the short run, but in Molly's case it was not working in the long run, and in truth had, from the beginning, been helping only a little.

Why after more than a year and a half of stomach acid–reducing medication was she still irritated? This was the important question. Her medical treatment had been thorough and consistent. There were no other symptoms of infection, such as an elevated white-blood-cell count (other than in her esophagus) or fever.

ALLERGY VERSUS INTOLERANCE

Could the underlying cause of Molly's misery be an allergy? Possibly. However, allergic reactions mean the presence of eosinophils, a type of white blood cell that causes irritating symptoms like itching and asthma. Other types of white cells respond to infections and irritations. According to her blood work, Molly did not have eosinophils in her blood, which is why the GI specialist had not recommended that she see an allergist. She did have white blood cells in her esophogus, which remained suspicious and was the first clue.

Although the specialist had ruled out allergies, I felt Molly's symptoms might still be an allergic reaction to something. Why? Because the immune systems of children two and under are still underdeveloped, they do not reliably produce eosinophils, which makes confirming allergies with a blood test unreliable. If the test results are positive, there is an allergy for sure, but a negative test does not reveal much of anything. Your child still may or may not suffer from an allergy, and there is no clear way to know if the result is a false negative or a true negative.

I began following the other clues, one of which was the fact that Molly did not have an infection. She certainly had not swallowed a Tinkertoy or mulch. She barely put food in her mouth, so her physical irritation was unlikely to have been caused by the ingestion of a foreign object.

I had another question: Why would food back up into the throat rather than move through her body and bother her intestines? If a substance is irritating, the body tries to expel the offender, like a watchful bouncer at a bar. The digestive tract is one long tube, so there are only two directions the offending substance can be sent: up and out or down and out. The normal direction is down and out, so the potential irritant has to be mighty annoying to be sent back the way it came. Molly had reflux, not diarrhea or stomach cramps, which meant that the problematic substances were being bounced upward.

The body chooses the route up versus down for two main reasons. For children under age two, the muscle tone around the stomach muscles has not developed enough to keep the tummy shape stable and pressure off the LES. The reason most spitting up stops on its own by age one is that children are usually walking by then and have developed their abdominal muscles enough to hold the shape of their belly so it does not put excessive pressure on the opening. Though children can have structural abnormalities, congenital defects, or other physical development problems that affect the normal shape or operation of the stomach, they are relatively rare.

The second reason for reflux symptoms is that a food can irritate the gut lining, causing the stomach to want to get rid of it. This can be an allergic or a nonallergic reaction. Remember, allergies are histamine driven. Histamine is an irritating substance that causes itching and swelling very soon (within two hours) after exposure. As mentioned before, eosinophils are the white blood cells that are activated by allergens. Upon activation, a number of substances are released that cause the tissue irritation (runny nose, itching) we have come to know and associate with allergies. If the eosinophils are not elevated and there is no itching or swelling, the reaction is considered nonallergic—but remember, in children under age two the reactions may not be clear-cut. Finding nonallergic food sensitivities is rarely a simple, straightforward process, because the reactions can be caused by numerous mechanisms, many of which are not understood. What causes a person to get tired or have

> Children *can* outgrow reactions, but time is not the cure for *all* allergies and sensitivities.

stomach pain from eating a food they are reacting to? Nobody knows for sure, but scientists suspect a group of obscure, unstable chemicals called cytokines. Though nonallergic food reactions/sensitivities are as common as, if not more common than, histamine reactions, they are often missed due to lack of accurate lab tests. The best strategy for finding food irritants is to eliminate the suspected dietary item and observe the result.

Based on both my observations and her mom's account of her developmental history, Molly's muscles were well developed. She sat up and walked on time and showed no signs of physical developmental delays. My best guess was, therefore, explanation number two: an irritant. And since we knew Molly was not eating very much, in fact almost nothing except the high-protein drink her pediatrician had recommended, I decided to take a closer look at the supplement's contents. Its primary ingredient was casein, the principal milk-based protein found in most cow-based dairy products. Casein is potentially the most difficult food in the human diet to digest.

The irritant could very well be dairy protein, since it was her main food and had been, in some form, since the GERD started.

I knew what we needed to do right away: Remove the possible irritant and help Molly heal her aggravated gut lining. Cow casein is complicated to digest, which is why it is "pre-" digested or partially broken down (hydrolyzed) in infant formulas. Even predigested, intolerance to it is one of the most common reasons for reflux in infants. Molly was a toddler, but I suspected she had not outgrown her reaction. Children *can* outgrow reactions, but time is not the cure for *all* allergies and sensitivities. Parents and doctors often cling to the hope that reactions are being outgrown even when clear evidence, as in this case, disputes the notion. Instead, Molly's situation had been muddied by many symptoms and medication trials. Now we suspected why she could not stop reflux medicine without worsening symptoms—the aggravator was still in the diet. Further, no medicine was strong enough to ameliorate the constant irritation. The situation was analogous to continuously picking at a scab with one hand while applying a bandage with the other. Hence, even on the medicine, eating was uncomfortable.

Molly's mother was nervous about removing dairy-based foods, believing her daughter would jump from mild malnutrition to full-blown starvation. Worrying her mother further was the fact that Molly didn't like solid food in general. Despite the ministrations of an eating therapist, her chronic pain and low interest in food had stalled her eating development at the baby-food stage. Nobody knew if she could not or would not eat more age-appropriate foods. We needed a healthy nondairy drink she would accept. I explained to Molly's mother that there were several possible ways to feed Molly safely:

1. Commercial formulas made from proteins other than casein, such as whey, soy, or goat's milk protein-based formulas

2. Formulas made from casein that are more predigested than regular formula, such as Alimentum and Nutramigen

3. Highly sophisticated formulas for severely reactive children that use free-form amino acids (the building blocks of protein) that are made in a laboratory, such as Neocate or EleCare

The Pros and Cons of Formula Alternatives

FORMULA SUBSTITUTE	PROS	CONS
Soy	Inexpensive; easy to get	Not recommended because of too much cross sensitivity and the use of GMO soy (see page 250)
Goat	Goat casein is similar to human	Not currently available in the U.S.; goat milk alone is not sufficient for children under age 1; may have some cross sensitivity
Whey	Inexpensive; easy to get	May still be irritating because whey is a milk protein
Super-predigested casein-based formulas (Alimentum, Nutramigen)	Less expensive than some other options; easily available	Smell awful; older infants tend to refuse; contain corn, which may be an irritant
Amino acid formulas (Neocate, EleCare)	Very low reactivity	Extremely hard on the pocketbook; bitter undertaste; contain corn, another potential irritant
Kelly's Yummy Cow-Free "Milk"	Only alternative when others fail; meets standards for most nutrients (except vitamin C) according to the National Infant Formula Act	Not laboratory tested

4. A carefully designed homemade recipe that includes rice or almond milk, coconut milk, and a special rice protein developed by yours truly that I call Kelly's Yummy Cow-Free "Milk"

There are pros and cons to each of these choices (see "The Pros and Cons of Formula Alternatives" on the facing page), and after carefully considering all of the options, I decided that my recipe might work for Molly. The one choice I tell all parents to avoid when dealing with potential milk sensitivity is soy formula because of the high cross sensitivity between soy and milk protein. About half of the children who react to

KELLY'S YUMMY COW-FREE "MILK" RECIPE

14 oz. calcium-fortified rice or almond milk

2 oz. unsweetened coconut milk—the kind that's high in fat and comes in a can, not coconut water

One scoop of Metagenics Ultracare for Kids (a predigested rice protein–based drink mix developed for kids with allergies). This product is available online.

Although I try to avoid recommending specific products and instead describe the desired characteristics, there is no substitute product for Ultracare for Kids, made by Metagenics, in my recipe. Do not use other protein powders. The dietary needs of babies are precise, so milk substitutes must be nutritionally complete.

RECIPE ADJUSTMENT TIPS: If you are using rice milk and your child gets constipated, substitute almond milk (with your doctor's okay), or reduce the rice milk to 13 ounces and increase the coconut milk to 3 ounces, or add some prune juice.

IMPORTANT WARNINGS: Unfortified rice and almond milk are not suitable milk substitutes and should not be given to children under age four. These "milks" have very little protein, few nutrients, and not enough fat to be considered nutritious. Think of them as similar to juice.

Talk to your health care practitioner before substituting this recipe for infant formula. Do not use this with infants under two years of age without medical supervision. Consulting a knowledgeable medical professional is recommended for all children when making major dietary adjustments.

This recipe is low in vitamin C, so make sure there are other sources of it in your child's diet or add it as a supplement.

cow's milk also react to soy milk. Some of them react to soy even more. Because of this phenomenon, parents often believe food and formula reactions are not causing the spitting up. After all, they switched from milk-based to soy formula, and their child was no better.

You may wonder whether there is any harm in trying soy formula, knowing it may not help. There isn't, but bear in mind that the chances of success are the same as flipping a coin. Those are not good enough odds if your child is suffering. Further, soy as a major protein source in the diet is becoming more and more controversial, so even if it "works," do you want a child consuming that much soy?

Goat's milk–based formula is an option, but there is also some cross sensitivity between cow's and goat's milk. All mammal milk contains casein, but the structure of the casein is different, depending on which animal produced it. Goat casein is more similar to human casein than cow casein is to human casein, which is why goat's milk is generally easier for humans to tolerate than cow's milk.

Molly was so miserable that we switched to Kelly's Yummy Cow-Free "Milk" cold turkey and hoped she would like it. She did, which isn't always the case. With children who are attached to their formula or milk, we sometimes make their new drink with three-quarters milk and one-quarter of the new dairy-free choice and change them over gradually.

The initial results were promising. Within days, Molly's appetite picked up and the irritation in her stomach and general discomfort were reduced. Now we

> The main benefits of consuming probiotics are enhanced immune functioning and better digestion.

needed to add nutrients to heal the intestinal lining. Just because you remove the nails in the driveway does not mean your car tires get better. Repair is necessary. There are many excellent nutritional products available for healing the gut. We used two with Molly: probiotics and zinc carnosine.

Probiotics are good bacteria. We all have good bacteria lining the insides of our GI tracts. They are an important part of balanced intestinal function. There are hundreds of studies attesting to their feats, but if you don't have time to read technical papers, you can hear all about them on television commercials for yogurt. "Strengthens your body's defenses," says one. "Regulates your digestive tract," heralds another. Yogurt naturally contains good bacteria, usually a *Lactobacillus* strain, but some manufacturers add extra. There is enough convincing evidence about the benefits of probiotics that the Food and Drug Administration allows companies to make general statements about their properties when the levels are significant. The main benefits of consuming good bacteria are enhanced immune functioning and better digestion. Much of the immune system operates around the digestive tract, because after the lungs, the mouth (and by extension the gut) is the easiest place for bad bugs to enter the body.

One way probiotics help the immune system is by improving the integrity of the gastrointestinal lining. Molly had plenty of irritation and needed plenty of healing there. She was going to be off dairy products, so the natural sources of good bacteria in most people's diets (mainly yogurt) were going to be unavailable. There are some fruit-, soy-, and coconut-based fermented drinks that contain probiotics, but even if Molly agreed to consume them, the amount of bacteria they contain would not be sufficient to heal her tummy.

Dozens of companies have conveniently packaged various

NUTRITION DETECTIVE PRINCIPLE #5

If your child has stomach pain, look first at what he or she is eating or drinking.

The vast majority of the children with reflux I have seen who do not have low muscle tone can be helped by removing the irritating foods from their diets. Sometimes, several types of foods need to be removed, more testing needs to be done, or we have to invoke the dreaded "trial and terror," where we have to guess based on history because the tests are not helping. But one of the safest ways to address reflux is to eliminate the most common irritant: casein.

strains of helpful bacteria in capsules or as powders. Drug and nutrient supplement manufacturers produce different proprietary blends of bugs, and all claim that their particular recipe is the best. Luckily, there are many excellent products to choose from. For Molly I chose a refrigerated capsule that blends several good bugs, with an estimated total bacteria count of about ten billion. Her mom pulled apart one capsule per day and mixed it in her drink. (For a guide on how to choose a good probiotic, see page 126.)

The second healing substance I added was zinc carnosine. Zinc carnosine is a little known gut repair product that has been thought to improve gastric health, specifically, the stomach lining. Researchers in London tested this theory by administering a gut irritant to healthy volunteers and then checked to see if zinc carnosine worked better than a placebo to heal them. Yes, getting scientific information sometimes means doing nasty things to nice volunteers. The volunteers were found to have guts that healed better when they took zinc carnosine in a "dose-dependent manner." In other words, the higher the dose, the faster the healing. Zinc carnosine comes in a chewable tablet and a pressed pill. Because Molly could not chew up a pill, we crushed the chewable to make it easier. She was only two years old, so we used just one pill per day for two months.

Eliminating dairy, substituting a healthy alternative, and adding two healing substances improved Molly's appetite almost immediately, but she had to reduce her reflux medicine little by little to avoid a rebound effect. Because there is very little stomach acid production when strong reflux medication is taken, time is needed to build up the stomach lining to protect it from a sudden acid infusion. Cutting the medicine down slowly allows the acid levels to slowly increase. Her stomach was not accustomed to holding a full component of stomach acid, so with the permission of her doctor, her mom reduced the medicine over the course of a few months.

Naturally, eating more food meant more weight gain, and slowly Molly started to put on the pounds. Once the pain was gone, she no longer needed a feeding therapist and taught herself to manipulate food in her mouth as most children do.

Her doctor was impressed with her dramatic improvement and wanted to revisit the possibility of an allergy. Was the culprit a real allergy or did Molly just have a strong reaction to dairy? The doctor retested Molly's blood directly for allergies, because now that she was over two years old, the test would be more accurate. This time Molly tested positive for an allergy to milk, but it's important to know that she could have had the same symptoms and not tested positive. If the allergy test had been negative, it would have changed nothing. Dairy often causes strong reactions that cannot be classified as allergies. However, Molly's mother was glad the doctor was so thorough and secretly glad to be able to document the source of her problems. Most parents never get confirmation of their suspicions through clear test results. (See page 92 for more on the inaccuracies of testing.)

Is Your Child's Reflux Caused by a Food Irritant?

When trying to determine whether or not your baby or young child's reflux (or GERD) is caused by a food intolerance, ask yourself the following questions:

☐ Was or is your child fussy or colicky after three months of age?

☐ Has your child been on reflux medicine for more than three months?

☐ If you try to take your child off the medicine, does he or she regress immediately?

☐ Did you have trouble finding a formula that suited your child? Were you advised to switch from breast-feeding to formula? (I have no idea why this ridiculous advice is given, but it is common.)

☐ Does your child have other signs of irritation such as constipation, loose stools, skin rashes, asthma, or frequent illnesses?

☐ Is your child with reflux older than two?

☐ Does your child have bad breath or burp excessively?

☐ Does your child have little interest in eating?

If you answered yes to two or more of these questions, read on.

What to Do

Responding to your child's reflux depends on a number of factors, primarily his or her age, as well as the degree of his reactiveness to casein or soy. Here are some ideas to discuss with your pediatrician that might help get your child off medicine for good.

If your child is twelve months or younger:

1. Removing potential irritants, usually from formula, is the most important consideration. However, there are physical positions that help take pressure off the baby's LES. Doctors recommend keeping the baby in a vertical position after eating, because sitting upright puts less pressure on the LES so it can keep the stomach contents in the stomach. A baby's sleeping position can also be adjusted. Children without GERD should sleep on their backs or on their sides propped by a firm bolster, but some doctors recommend that babies with reflux sleep on their stomachs. You may want to discuss sleep positions with your doctor, because there may be an increase in instances of sudden infant death syndrome when babies sleep on their tummies. You also want to take extra precautions, such as removing pillows and using a firm mattress.

2. Talk to your pediatrician about commercial formulas made from proteins other than casein, such as whey or soy. Consider the pros and cons of trying one or skipping to the next step.

3. Try a formula made from casein that is very highly predigested, such as Alimentum or Nutramigen. This may be more diffficult if your child is older than seven or eight months because of the stronger taste of this type of formula.

4. Try a highly sophisticated laboratory-made formula for severely reactive children that uses free-form amino acids (the building blocks of protein), such as Neocate or EleCare.

5. Keep in close communication with your health care provider so adjustments can be made if the formula is not working.

For children over age one:

1. Consider removing dairy foods from the diet. Discontinue milk, ice cream, cheese, yogurt, and pudding. Do not worry about butter or the small amounts of dairy products that may be cooked into, say, a piece of bread at first. If the child turns out to be highly reactive (like Molly), you can go back later and take out the foods with minor dairy components.

2. If your child likes to drink milk, consider goat's milk or Kelly's Yummy Cow-Free "Milk." Plain rice and almond milk are not suitable milk substitutes on their own, and should not be given to children under age four. These "milks" have very little protein, few nutrients, and not enough fat to be considered nutritious. They need to be fortified with fat, protein, and other nutrients to be close to equivalent to milk in nutritional value.

   If you are afraid your child will never drink something new, try mixing Kelly's Yummy Cow-Free "Milk" or goat's milk with cow's milk in equal proportions for the first week. Then completely remove the cow's milk the second week.

   Children who drink two cups per day of Kelly's Yummy Cow-Free "Milk" should not need additional calcium. If your child refuses the milk substitute or you choose not to use it, the child will need 800 to 1,000 milligrams of calcium per day. Give half the amount in the morning and half later in the day for maximum absorption.

3. Make a plan with your doctor for slowly reducing reflux medicine as symptoms improve.

CHAPTER 6

The Girl Whose Tummy Always Hurt

A S PARENTS, WE ARE ALL familiar with stomach complaints. "I have a bellyache, Dad." "Why won't my stomach stop hurting?" "I want to stay home—my tummy still bothers me." These complaints can be so frequent that we often wonder whether they're true or are actually a case of the Monday-morning school blues. It can be confusing. Kids often somatize their feelings, especially fears and nervousness, and experience difficult emotions in their bodies. Abdominal pain is a great reason to skip a math test, especially if a child feels as if she might throw up. And for many of us, some math tests are upsetting enough to induce digestive distress. However, "stress" or "anxiety" is too often the fallback diagnosis when medical problems cannot clearly explain certain symptoms, such as the all-too-familiar tummy ache.

Luckily, most parents have good instincts about when to accept anxiety as the cause of their kids' distress and when to keep digging for another cause of the problem, suspecting that something more physiological might lie behind the chronic stomach complaints. Ellen was one of these savvy moms: savvy and busy. As a single mom, she spent every free moment after work chauffeuring her two teenage daughters to appointments and team sports activities. Most of the appointments were with medical specialists trying to figure out why her younger daughter, Shane, was constantly sick to her stomach. A less determined mom would have long ago thrown in the towel and sent Shane to a psychologist, but not Ellen. She knew something was physically wrong with her otherwise strong and even-tempered daughter. Together, let's follow the clues to get to the bottom of Shane's near-constant bellyache.

SHANE AND HER BAD TUMMY

Fourteen-year-old Shane had been grouchy about her stomach for years and felt that she just couldn't take it anymore. A constant dull ache regularly expanded to debilitating sharp pain. On those days she would stay home from school and lie in bed. By the time she came to my office, along with her mother and older sister, Whitney, Shane had seen four gastroenterologists and had received multiple diagnoses, including irritable bowel syndrome, gastritis, and GERD (reflux). The specialists had prescribed a large array of medications, none of which had reduced her pain or explained her discomfort. The pain had started when she was about seven years old and was a daily occurrence, along with frequent vomiting, loose stools alternating with constipation, and asthma. To treat the pain, asthma, and reflux, her doctor had put Shane on several medicines, which she took dutifully but with no relief.

Shane was outgoing and wanted to be an engaged and busy high schooler, but she could barely show up each morning. Her low energy level limited her participation in after-school activities and social outings with friends. Determined to do some of the things she liked in spite of exhaustion and chronic pain, Shane tried out for and made a travel soccer team. After games, she sometimes had to lie on the ground until she felt well enough to walk to the car.

By the time Shane got to my office, her mother was comfortable with meeting new professionals and got down to business quickly. Ellen had spared no expense in seeking out top specialists who had ruled out celiac disease (see "Gluten Intolerance Versus Celiac Disease" on page 92), ulcers, food allergies, and inflammatory bowel disease. Shane had been scoped from both ends (endoscopy and colonoscopy–see "The Scoop on Scopes" on page 72) with the only clear findings indicating reflux and gastritis (inflammation of the lining of the stomach). After taking a detailed history of Shane's health and listening to all the diagnoses, which included asthma along with the GI-related ones, plus Shane's less-than-satisfactory reactions to the medicines, I realized that I was going to have to treat these diagnoses as a starting point. I had a strong hunch that they were not the final word for understanding what was going on with Shane. In other words, if the diagnoses were accurate, her treatment should have been more successful.

The fact that Shane had received more than one diagnosis pointed to the possibility that something not yet uncovered might be the key to all the various symptoms: the constant pain, the diarrhea alternating with constipation, the reflux, and perhaps even the asthma. I looked around me at the three related females sitting in my office. Maybe they harbored some clues? Shane maintained a normal weight, but her mother and older sister were obese.

"Does anyone else have tummy troubles?" I inquired.

"Oh, yes–I have constant discomfort and diarrhea, but not nearly as bad as Shane," Ellen volunteered. Shane's sister then revealed that she too had milder but persistent stomach issues. They were a sour-stomach trio, with Shane having the dubious honor of being first violin. Because looking at her alone had not helped the specialists unravel her issues, I decided to consider the patterns within the whole group.

Ellen was a veteran of medical office visits and had come prepared with Shane's food diary. Suspecting that her whole family's diet needed a tune-up, she had decided to be prepared, and brought her own and Whitney's food records as well. Shane's daily log consisted of muffins or bagels plus a piece of fruit for breakfast; a peanut butter and jelly sandwich, cookies, and water for lunch; another bagel or English muffin for a snack; and Gatorade, cookies, and pasta, with an occasional hamburger, salad, or chicken tender thrown in for dinner.

The vast majority of the foods on this list were wheat based:

- muffins
- bagels
- pasta
- cookies
- bread for sandwiches

The same was true of Ellen and Whitney's diet: All three of them were eating similar foods, with Ellen and Whitney eating larger quantities. Given the fact that none of the other diagnoses Shane had been given had gotten to the root of her stomach problems, I had a hunch that her stomach pain, vomiting, and other symptoms were actually a reaction to gluten, the protein in wheat that made up the bulk of her meals.

When asked about her symptoms, Ellen revealed that she, too, had reflux. She confessed, "Reflux medicine does help me, though I am often bloated anyway. I was hoping Shane would get at least some relief."

Within one family we have these consistent symptoms:

- stomach pain
- reflux
- constipation
- bloat (gas)
- loose stools

This is a fairly complete list of the gastrointestinal symptoms associated with gluten intolerance. There are other systemic symptoms of gluten intolerance, including rashes, joint pain, headaches, and uncontrolled appetite (see page 101 for a complete list of the many and varied symptoms of gluten intolerance), but the tummy ones are sufficient to point to gluten as the culprit.

In the previous chapter, Molly had reflux, another source of stomach pain, that came from an intolerance of dairy products. What is the

Your Food Diary: An Important Tool

I always ask my clients to bring in a record of everything they have eaten for several days. A food diary is more helpful than asking people to tell you what they eat, because people often think they are eating better than they actually are. If asked what we eat, most of us report what we mean to eat, not what we actually put in our mouths. Our food memories and estimations can be way off if we are not writing down what we eat at the time.

The best way to keep a food diary is to jot down what your child is eating in a small notebook or handheld computer several times during the day. If your memory is especially good, you can write it all down at night. Do not write three days' worth at one time, because selective memory will start to creep in and distort the accuracy of the results. Estimate quantity as best you can without measuring unless instructed by your health care practitioner to do otherwise.

difference between these two cases? The biggest difference is in the diet. Molly consumed dairy products almost exclusively, whereas Shane's intake was heavily balanced toward gluten, so I picked the food that was most prevalent in each of their diets. In addition, Molly's symptoms started before age one and the introduction of gluten-based foods. However, if a child eats a good amount of both, I first look for the presence of one of the other symptoms associated with gluten intolerance, such as headaches. If that fails, I reexamine the timing of the symptoms and introduction of foods. The older the child is when the symptoms appear, the more likely I am to blame gluten. But if no other clues cause me to suspect one over another, I ask the parents to make a guess and go with that for the purposes of the elimination trial.

I suggested that Shane try a gluten-free diet, explaining quickly that there are many more gluten-free foods available now than there were even just a few years ago—and many taste great! (See "A Sample Gluten-Free Daily Diet" on page 97.) I also suggested that because the entire family suffered from stomach issues, they might want to try a gluten-free diet together, knowing that Shane would have a much easier time making the transition if she was not the only person eating in this new and different way. Ellen had long suspected that pasta and bread were causing her to bloat, and because both she and Shane's sister had weight issues, she figured the worst that would happen is that they would lose a few pounds. I knew the odds of Shane following a gluten-free diet were going to be much higher if she had her family's support, and perhaps the others would benefit, too.

TROUBLE IN A BREAD BASKET

Gluten is a complicated protein that is found in all wheat and also in some other grains such as barley, spelt, and rye. Most people do not think of bread or pasta as major dietary protein sources, and they are correct. The small amount of gluten protein in wheat is important because it is what gives bread its unique spongy texture. There are many families of gluten. Oats, for example, contain gluten from a different family than wheat gluten, and the slight difference in the two glutens' structures allows oats to be tolerated by many people who are sensitive to wheat gluten.

In medicine, the classic illness associated with gluten intolerance is celiac disease (see "Gluten Intolerance Versus Celiac Disease," page 92). When celiac disease is ruled out, as it was via endoscopy in Shane's case, doctors tend to assume that gluten is not the problem. This black-and-white thinking limits their ability to see how irritating gluten can be even when it is not causing celiac disease, which is a narrow, severe manifestation of gluten intolerance.

There is a corny old joke in medicine that goes like this: A man with a cold goes to see his doctor. "What seems to be the problem?" the physician asks.

"My nose won't stop running. I have a fever and my head hurts. This cold is making me miserable," the man moans. "What should I do?"

"My best advice is to take off all your clothes and stand in front of an open window," the doctor advises.

"But it's winter, and I will get pneumonia!" the man sputters.

"Yes, but that we can fix," the doctor proclaims triumphantly.

Of course, a real doctor would not make such a joke and instead would recommend palliative measures, but the point is that between a full-blown treatable illness and vibrant good health, there are a lot of vague and debilitating symptoms. Unfortunately, doctors can get stuck in a professional dilemma when the test results are negative or uncertain. They need evidence their colleagues will recognize and respect, but the patient wants concrete answers—now. Further, all tests have weaknesses, and some patients will fall through the cracks. When the symptoms and tests do not match, should the physician pick the closest diagnosis and treat, or hold off treatment and continue to pursue more and more obscure possibilities?

The fact that Shane's stomach was bothering her all the time was a clear symptom of gluten intolerance. It was also likely that she was intolerant of lactose (milk sugar), because most people who are gluten-intolerant lose the ability to digest lactose. More about that later.

GOING GLUTEN-FREE

Ellen agreed to put the entire family on an essentially gluten-free diet. Because Shane did not have celiac disease, we didn't have to be super-strict. Luckily for Shane and most people suffering from gluten intolerance, she needed to take out only those foods made with flour (e.g., bread, cereal, crackers, pasta, muffins, waffles and pancakes, pie crust, coated deep-fried items, and cookies). In most cities, major grocery store chains have sections that offer substitutes for products that contain gluten, including cake and pancake mixes, cookies, crackers, and pizza crust, demonstrating that both the awareness of the issue and the need for gluten-free products are much higher now.

The only food that is tough to replace is bread. The taste and texture of bread made with wheat flour is hard to reproduce. Indeed, what makes bread satisfying to eat is the unique texture gluten provides. The protein in gluten makes bread spongy. Breads without gluten tend to be either rubbery (like an old shoe) or crumbly. But as more and more creative bakers take on gluten-free cooking, bread choices are beginning to improve. One notably tasty gluten-free bread, according to a number of discriminating parents, is Deland's millet bread . A second contender is Udi's brand. Happily, there are many dedicated companies making excellent gluten-free products that will satisfy even the fussiest gourmet.

During the two-week trial period, I also asked Shane and the rest of her family to drink only lactose-free milk and to avoid ice cream. Lactose is the sugar contained in milk. Among dairy products, ice cream and milk contain the most lactose. The reason cheese and yogurt contain less is that most of the lactose is eaten by the bacteria used to ferment these foods. Lactase, the enzyme that breaks down milk sugar, is made at the edge of the intestinal lining. Its production is easily

GLUTEN INTOLERANCE VERSUS CELIAC DISEASE

Celiac disease (CD) is an autoimmune disease triggered by the ingestion of gluten, a protein found in wheat, barley, rye, and some other grains. The immune system attacks the gastrointestinal lining, resulting in a reduction in nutrient absorption. Autoimmune diseases can affect the entire body, and CD is associated with other problems such as immune deficiency and dermatitis herpetiformis, an itchy skin condition that goes away when gluten is removed. Nobody knows why eating gluten causes so many seemingly unrelated conditions such as chronic anemia, neurological problems, osteoporosis, joint pain, chronic fatigue, short stature, skin lesions, epilepsy, seizures, dementia, and cancer.

According to the Mayo Clinic, CD is on the rise. Its 2009 study published in *Gastroenterology* found that 1 in 100 people has celiac disease, making it four times more common now than it was in the 1950s. Further, it can take as long as seventeen years to diagnose. The study compared a sampling of blood taken from veterans from Warren Air Force Base between 1948 and 1954 with the blood of a sampling of people today. The comparison showed that more people are intolerant of gluten today than fifty years ago.

Although gluten intolerance has some of the same symptoms as CD, it does not present as an autoimmune gut-lining problem and is therefore not seen using endoscopy or found with a biopsy. The endoscopy is generally normal in cases of gluten sensitivity, although sometimes reflux

thrown off by the consumption of irritants, such as gluten. Once Shane's stomach calmed down and healed, she might be able to eat ice cream again, but until then, I did not want her to be irritated by lactose.

The result for Shane? Once she stopped eating gluten, all her stomach pains and bowel problems disappeared within a week. Her diet improved because she ate more chicken, fruit, and salad and did not automatically reach for an English muffin after school. After school she snacked on vegetables and hummus or grabbed a gluten-free protein bar if she was running off to soccer practice. Ellen took the girls food shopping, and they got more creative with their eating. Because she and Whitney wanted to lose weight, she did not substitute rice and potatoes very often for the pasta they often had for dinner but stuck to vegetables and meat. She bought gluten-free cookies and chips to pack in Shane's lunch.

---

can be found, as in Shane's case. Sensitivity is usually diagnosed by symptoms or sometimes with an anti-gliadin antibody blood test. This test is not specific for celiac disease but measures as many as three different immune responses to gluten. The immune system is not designed to fight food but is supposed to react to germs. An elevated immune response to gluten means the immune system is being led astray by gluten and not operating properly.

An endoscopy is the gold standard procedure used to diagnose CD. A gastroenterologist may order this test if the screening blood tests for CD are positive. CD blood screening tests, such as one that looks for endomysial antibodies, are not very accurate, because doctors and researchers have not yet figured out the exact cause or triggers for intolerance itself. But according to Dr. Peter Green, one of the world's top celiac disease experts, there is a reason why the average time it takes to get a CD diagnosis is eleven years: lousy tests. Although there are many other nonmainstream tests promising to identify gluten intolerance in stool or blood, their accuracy is also uncertain. One laboratory, that I will not name for the sake of politeness, finds gluten sensitivity in 80 percent of the samples. If I wanted a test result to "prove" that a child needed to go off gluten, I could use that lab, but that would be allowing the ends to justify the means at best, and unscrupulous at worst. So if you suspect that gluten is bothering your child, the best test remains an elimination trial: Take it out of the diet and see what happens.

WHEN YOU NEED TO BE SUPER-STRICT

For people who have full-blown celiac disease, ingesting even tiny amounts of gluten derivatives can cause a severe reaction or long-term damage. The damage can be done before the diagnosis is made, and the connection to eating gluten may not be obvious. A teenage girl with osteoporosis came to see me a number of years ago. She did not have stomach symptoms, but we discovered that the osteoporosis was caused by undiagnosed celiac disease. In addition to removing easy-to-see gluten-based flours from the diet, people with CD need to be careful of items such as commercial salad dressings, because for them starch additives (such as malt) are potential dietary bombs.

Finding hidden gluten can be complicated and time consuming. One child with celiac disease in my practice suddenly started having diarrhea, even though he hadn't made any changes to his diet. His highly intuitive mother suspected the potato chips she sometimes gave him, although the little boy had been eating the same brand for years. No wheat or starch derivatives were listed on the label, but she called the company to ask anyway. They denied using flour, but the mom was a pit bull (in the best sense of the word) and called three times. On the third try, she finally reached a knowledgeable person who confirmed that the company had started using flour at some point in production.

Teenagers have a reputation for being difficult, but Shane's dietary transformation was practically seamless. Her stomach improved so quickly that she had no desire to eat the offending foods and regulated herself without monitoring. If she cheated and had a piece of bread, the pain returned instantly. I have found that her reaction is common. Although most children need several weeks to adjust to the idea, most self-regulate like Shane once they know which foods to avoid. Until then, if they are unsure, they ask the adults around them if the food contains gluten before eating it.

Having the rest of the family on the diet always helps, especially in the beginning. Unfortunately, getting or keeping every member of the family on the program is not always possible or, in other cases, necessary. Shane's entire family benefited from the diet, so in her case the situation was optimal. Ellen's stomach bloat went away, and her other symptoms greatly diminished on the diet. Whitney also improved and started to lose weight. But here comes the "people do the darndest things" part: Only Shane stayed on the diet. Shane's mother and sister decided they liked pasta too much and could live with their symptoms and extra weight. Ellen continued to provide gluten-free food for Shane but collapsed under pressure from Whitney to buy bagels, slipping back into old habits outside the house by the second month. I looked at Shane after Ellen explained the current state of affairs. She looked uncomfortable but determined. "Are you going to be all right?" I asked. She just shrugged. I rightly took that as a yes.

WHAT EXACTLY IS GLUTEN ANYWAY, AND WHY IS IT SO HARD TO AVOID?

Gluten is a nonspecific term derived from the Latin word for "glue." Glue to gluten—no big surprises there. Most cookbooks describe gluten as the protein that makes the dough in bread and other baked goods stretchy and yummy. Gluten is not one protein but a type of protein. In wheat, the specific gluten is gliadin. Rye has secalin, and barley, hordein. There are loads of gluten substances and cousins. Hordein, gliadin, and secalin sound more like a group of cute Southern belles, but they are closely related, and all have to be avoided by those with celiac disease and gluten sensitivity. Oats, on the other hand, also contain a gluten called avenin, but this particular gluten rarely bothers people with celiac disease. So, even though oats technically contain gluten, most gluten-sensitive people can tolerate it.

WHAT YOU CAN EAT ON A GLUTEN-FREE DIET

- good old grains: rice, corn
- fun new grains: millet, amaranth, wild rice, quinoa
- potatoes
- any meat, vegetable, fruit, nut, seed, dairy product (although liquid milk and ice cream bothers many people intolerant to gluten)
- legumes (kidney beans, black beans, pinto beans, etc.)

No wonder food labeling has been mired in confusion. Are oats labeled "gluten-free" really without gluten? They cannot be, because oats contain gluten. They would be more accurately labeled "wheat-gluten–free." Some oat companies use flour or other starch in the processing, and that is a problem for celiacs. Long, consistent lobbying efforts have attempted to clarify labeling with only mixed success.

Label reading gets worse when vague terms such as *modified food starch* are used. The source could be corn, tapioca, potato, wheat, or some laboratory-derived mystery starch (with the exception of wheat, all safe for the gluten-free). If it is not specified, the consumer is forced to err on the side of avoidance or spend long hours on the phone with pleasant but generally unhelpful food company representatives.

Here is a beginning list of groups and companies that specialize in gluten-free living:

- Celiac.com (www.celiac.com). General comprehensive support to help people live a healthy, gluten-free life.

- *Living Without* magazine (www.livingwithout.com). Dedicated to supporting those on elimination diets of all types, including gluten.

- Celiac Disease Foundation (www.celiac.org). National organization that represents the celiac community.

- *Gluten-Free Living* magazine (www.glutenfreeliving.com).

- University of Maryland Center for Celiac Research (www.celiaccenter .org). Supports research and increases awareness about celiac disease.

- Children's Digestive Health and Nutrition Foundation (www.celiac health.org). Informational website on various digestive ailments, including celiac disease, run by pediatric gastroenterologists.

- What? No Wheat? Enterprises (www.whatnowheat.com). Publishes gluten-free educational materials, provides links to support groups and gluten-free bakeries.

- Allergy Grocer (www.allergygrocer.com). Commercial site that sells gluten-free flours and products. One of many, many sites.

CHARLOTTE'S QUANDARY

Let's look at another example of how gluten intolerance manifests. Charlotte, a ten-year-old girl of average height, was slightly chubby around the middle. Her mother brought her in to see me because she was worried. For the past few months, Charlotte had woken up complaining about stomach pain and headaches every day. When I asked Charlotte how often she thought she felt bad, she responded, "Once in a while." Of course, parents and children often experience the same situation differently. This is a common human experience best summed up by a scene in an old Woody Allen movie. Someone asks a couple how often they have sex. "Hardly ever," the man laments. "Constantly," the woman complains.

A Sample Gluten-Free Daily Diet

	BEGINNER'S ALL-AMERICAN	ADVANCED HEALTH-ENHANCING
BREAKFAST	• eggs • home fries • fruit	• oatmeal with 1 tablespoon pumpkin seeds, 1 tablespoon sliced almonds, 1 tablespoon dried cherries or raisins, and ½ banana topped with yogurt
LUNCH	• turkey-and-cheese roll-up • carrot sticks • baked potato chips • grapes	• lentil soup • small salad • Nut Thins or other gluten-free crackers • clementine
DINNER	• chicken and rice • creamed corn • salad • frozen yogurt	• wild-caught salmon • brown rice • broccoli • goat cheese with a side of grapes

I thought it was important to find out if the mom was over-reporting or Charlotte was feeling defensive and underestimating. We went through the previous week day by day. Charlotte admitted that she had had a headache and tummy ache during a Saturday event and that the discomfort persisted all of Sunday. Her mom then chimed in that Charlotte had stayed home from school twice in the previous week. They also recalled a day when Charlotte had thrown herself on the ground, overcome by discomfort and agitation. Faced with this now-remembered evidence, Charlotte confessed, "I guess I felt bad every day. But I try not to think about it."

It's hard to get details from kids Charlotte's age about how pain feels. Charlotte was not necessarily in denial about her head and tummy aches—it's more likely that she didn't want to be seen as "the girl who is always sick," which is typical of most tween girls who don't want anything to make them stand apart or seem different from their peers. "It must be hard to feel bad most of the time," I sympathized.

Relaxing slightly, Charlotte admitted that that very morning she had woken up with both a headache and a stomachache. I asked her what she'd eaten the night before; she'd had a grilled cheese sandwich and a glass of milk for dinner. Most nights she ate pasta with butter. She said she thought eating bread and pasta would "calm down my tummy."

I asked some more questions:

1. Did Charlotte have constipation? No.
2. Diarrhea? No.

The only clue other than Charlotte's near-constant tummy ache and her headache was that she also happened to be a picky eater. As Charlotte and her mother described her general diet, it was clear that it was restricted mostly to pasta, cereal, bread, milk, and cheese.

So here were the clues:

1. near constant tummy ache
2. headache
3. diet made up of mostly gluten- and dairy-based foods

By this point, an intrepid nutrition detective will recognize several of the symptoms from the gluten-sensitivity symptom list. Shane also had the near-constant tummy ache from gluten, but Molly from the last chapter had pain from dairy. Charlotte's restricted diet had both gluten- and dairy-based foods. The irritant was not going to be peanut butter because she never ate it! If the pain is an everyday occurrence, the irritant has to be something eaten every day, which in Charlotte's case meant gluten or casein.

But I didn't think it was casein. Why? First, the symptoms were recent (they had started in the last several months). If children had problems with dairy when they were babies, symptoms sometimes reappear later in a different form. Charlotte did not have a history of formula or dairy intolerance. Second, she did not have constipation (a more common dairy symptom) but did have headaches (a more common gluten symptom). Children can get headaches from dairy and constipation from gluten, but these scenarios are rare.

For this reason, I thought Charlotte should start with a gluten-free diet. This news made her very upset. Her mother was trying to be supportive and enthusiastic, saying, "This is going to be fun!" I told the mom that Charlotte might go through a short "withdrawal" period as she adjusted to the new diet. Her mouth sagged. "What exactly do you mean by *withdrawal?*"

"Well, it's not as bad as going to the Betty Ford Clinic," I ventured, feeling guilty for ruining the rosy picture she was trying to paint for Charlotte. "But some children crave the food they are reacting to, a bit like an older person craving cigarettes or alcohol. Consequently, there can be a few touchy days when the desire for the food is all-consuming. It passes quickly," I assured, "but do not get discouraged if there are some meltdowns and tears. Things might seem a little worse before they get better." (For information on improving the diet of a picky eater, read about the E.A.T. program described on page 52.)

If the pain subsides, most picky eaters come through this transition into a new eating plan more open and amenable to trying new foods. As with Shane, I recommended that Charlotte avoid lactose-heavy milk

NUTRITION DETECTIVE
PRINCIPLE #6

Food intolerance is not always all or nothing.

A person can react poorly to a food without having a full-blown disease or intolerance. For example, a child can be gluten-intolerant without having celiac disease or can be lactose-intolerant without being allergic to milk. Some people can consume small amounts of the troublesome food without experiencing symptoms, whereas others will react to even a tiny amount. However, just because small amounts are tolerated does not mean the suspicious food is safe at any quantity. When testing for food sensitivity, we take the suspected food out of a person's diet completely for several weeks to reduce the number of variables and establish a baseline. Once we know how the person does without the food in the diet, we add a little back and see how he or she does. Ultimately, by trial and error, we establish a tolerance point.

and ice cream, but not cheese and yogurt. Now Charlotte was turning an unflattering shade of green. "No milk, either," she gasped.

Lactose intolerance is probably the most common everyday cause of stomach distress, especially when burping and gas is involved. As with Shane, I was afraid that the damage the gluten had done to Charlotte's digestive lining had disrupted her lactase production (the enzyme that breaks down lactose). Most people with celiac disease lose the ability to digest milk sugar, and the gluten-intolerant often share the same fate. Lactose is what makes milk sweet. The reason milk is sweet and plain yogurt is not is that good bacteria turn milk into yogurt by eating all the milk sugar. Without much lactose, yogurt tastes tangy. It is also easier to digest because the good bacteria (probiotics or bugs) help the digestive tract.

All of this boils down to you being able to tell your kids with confidence, "Eat your bugs—they are good for you!" It is hard to tell children they cannot have their favorite foods—there have been many times when I've felt like the Grinch who stole Christmas—but the consolation prize is that so many of them feel better. After a few days off gluten, milk, and ice cream, Charlotte's tummy and head were almost completely better. But she was discouraged. The mean nutritionist had taken away her favorite foods! She wanted to know if or when she could add some of them back.

"CHEATING"

Can people with gluten intolerance ever start eating foods with gluten in them again, and if so, when and how much? There is no easy answer to that. It is all individual trial and error. Generally, people with gluten intolerance cannot go back to the average American diet, which is heavily gluten based; however, some kids can handle a sandwich here, a crouton there. Shane gets stomach pain immediately when she cheats, but that could change years down the road. After several weeks on the diet, Charlotte was able to handle some milk and ice cream without feeling bad. Both children were so much more comfortable not eating the foods that were making them sick that they adjusted well to their new way of eating, though Charlotte needed more time—about eight weeks in total—before the issue of missing gluten faded. In my experience, children under age twelve adapt well and quickly to dietary changes, unless they are dealing with other developmental issues alongside their dietary one. All bets are off with teenagers and adults. They are much more unpredictable.

Is Your Child Sensitive to Gluten?

Check how many of the following symptoms suggesting gluten sensitivity apply to your child. I have indicated the symptoms that Shane and Charlotte had, but as you'll see, there are additional symptoms that we'll discuss in chapter 12.

☐ frequent cramping or stomach pain *(Shane and Charlotte)*

☐ extreme mood swings

☐ belligerent or oppositional behavior

☐ craving gluten-based foods in an almost druglike way

☐ a diet of mostly gluten-based foods *(Shane and Charlotte)*

☐ frequent loose stools or diarrhea or alternating loose stools and constipation *(Shane)*

☐ other family members with similar problems or a family history of celiac disease *(Shane)*

☐ older than age two, not overweight but has reflux *(Shane)*

☐ frequent, unexplained headaches *(Charlotte)*

☐ frequent, unexplained joint pain

☐ poor growth or bone loss

☐ excessive gas and bloat *(Charlotte)*

If your child has three or more of the symptoms listed above, there is a high likelihood that your child is intolerant of gluten.

What to Do

Below are some standard directions for how to do a gluten-free trial:

1. Eliminate gluten from your child's diet for one month. Remove all obvious candidates—bread, pasta, crackers, pancakes, cookies, and cakes—but do not worry about hidden ingredients at first.

2. Keep a record of what your child is eating and how he or she is feeling daily *while* doing the elimination trial. A calendar works well for this. The record will help spur your memory and identify potential problem areas.

3. If you need further support either because your child is a picky eater or because there are other issues, make an appointment with a health care practitioner experienced with gluten-free diets. This could be a gastroenterologist, nutritionist, nurse practitioner, or pediatrician. The important criterion is that they have experience with the gluten-free diet.

4. Minimize lactose (found in milk and ice cream) during the trial period. Once you determine whether gluten is a problem, add the lactose back and see if it is tolerated.

CHAPTER 7

The Case of the Boy Who Wouldn't Grow

A S PARENTS, ONE OF THE first ways we measure our children's development is with the growth chart. I'm sure you've heard other parents refer to what percentile their child is—and I'm not talking SATs. I'm talking inches and pounds. From the day they are born, we are told how our children are faring in terms of how they compare in weight and height with other children. After all, that is what a growth chart is—an average measure of the height and weight of a large number of children considered "typical," and most of us want a typical child.

Other charts exist for conditions known to have unique growth curves, such as Down syndrome, but most growth charts differentiate only in terms of sex, which is why there are separate charts for boys and girls. Although a growth chart can be a useful screening tool, it tells you only about your child's relative size, not how he got there or how to help him grow. I say it may be time to put aside the growth chart and instead look at the "what-the-child-is-eating" chart.

LIAM: WHEN SIZE MATTERS

Twelve-year-old Liam was small for his age. Really small. At twelve years old, he weighed seventy pounds and was 4 feet 6 inches tall, making him the smallest boy, by far, in his class.

For years, his parents had been concerned about Liam's small stature, but because he was consistently on "the growth chart" (though admittedly near the bottom), his pediatrician declared him "fine" and "following his own curve." He and the other specialists the family had consulted maintained that someone had to be at the bottom of the chart, so why not Liam? The boy was otherwise healthy and had a charming personality, so count your blessings, the experts advised. His parents and the rest of his family were of average height, so they felt like they were getting the brush-off.

Two years earlier, one endocrinologist had run a bone-age test. This is a noninvasive test that uses an X-ray of the wrist bone to estimate the age of the child. Obviously, the parent usually knows how old the child is, but the bone growth does not always keep pace with the chronological age of the child. If a ten-year-old child is the size of an eight-year-old, you want her bones' age to be eight. That way her size matches her bone age (not her chronological age) and she will likely be a "late bloomer."

Liam's bone age was close to his chronological age, so the endocrinologist predicted his adult height would be 5 feet 6 inches, plus or minus two inches. This final height is in the tenth percentile for males. "Hopefully, that will reassure him (and you) that he is normal!" the doctor wrote in a note to the mother. She was not reassured.

The last specialist, another endocrinologist, had reluctantly run blood tests to screen for growth hormone deficiency, but when Liam's levels were normal, the doctor told his parents to feed him more, saying that he would eventually grow. Liam's mother, Wendy, felt that cajoling Liam to eat was a full-time job, and she already had one of those. Besides, she had tried pestering him for years, and it was not working. He did not like constantly being pressured to eat, and she was not happy getting in touch with her inner nag. A family friend, who also happened to be a physician, intervened and suggested they come see me.

Formerly a bright student and engaging athlete, Liam was now literally being left on the sidelines. He struck me as a big personality stuffed into a miniature body. He was visibly unhappy when he arrived at my office, and it became quickly apparent that he was tired of being the cute little kid waiting for his body to catch up with his brain: He wanted to grow up. In the two years since the bone-age test, he had grown three inches and put

> Hunger represents one of our basic instincts for survival. If it's hampered or not operating, then something is definitely haywire in the body.

on four pounds. Although he had grown, the gain was so small that he had actually dropped from the tenth percentile on the growth chart to the fifth percentile. Of course, some kids and adults are naturally small in stature, but Liam was actually becoming smaller both in stature and in terms of his percentile—and I had to figure out why.

When I'm with preteens and older children who are facing issues that have been unsuccessfully but thoroughly evaluated, I often ask them what they think the problem is.

When I asked Liam this question, he replied, "I don't know. I try to eat as much as I can, but I am just not very hungry."

Liam had unwittingly revealed the first and ultimately critical clue to his lack of growth: He was rarely hungry.

This was important: Hunger represents one of our basic instincts for survival. If this primitive drive is hampered or not operating, then something is definitely haywire in the body. Liam did not have proper hunger instincts, and left to his own devices might have been even smaller than he was. His conscientious food-pushing parents had probably helped him get to the size he was, but they were doomed to failure if they were working against an underdeveloped appetite, a hunger drive gone awry. I knew I needed to pay attention to this clue.

My first step was to check for other physical symptoms that could distort the hunger signal. Stomach pains, certain medications, sleep issues, reflux, depression, and other conditions can all interfere with appetite. I fished around Liam's history by asking a ton of questions just to be sure nothing had been missed by previous professionals.

While we were reviewing their medical journey, Liam's mother, Wendy, quipped that she could not seem to get it just right. She was referring to Liam's older brother, who had problems on the other end of the spectrum and was on the edge of obesity. Wendy was living a twisted version of Goldilocks and the Three Bears—she had one child who was too big and one who was too little, but no child who was "just right." The fact that Liam's brother was overweight led me to believe that food availability was not an issue as it is in some households.

Many underweight adolescents complain that "there is nothing to eat in the house." Although some parents roll their eyes and counter with a description of an overflowing refrigerator and cupboards, others admit that their busy schedules do not allow them to shop for food often enough. There may be several days a week when the choices are limited, and some children would rather skip a snack or meal than eat peanut butter *again*. In this case, the problem is not financial poverty but time poverty. A glance at our society's increasingly overweight youngsters suggests that food availability is not a primary concern, but it remains a trouble spot for select populations.

Liam, however, lived in a food-friendly house, and in addition, there were no particular patterns of nutrient malabsorption in the family. (Sometimes a lack of growth or difficulty gaining or maintaining weight may be related to an inability to absorb nutrients. Liam had no digestive problems. His bowels functioned normally, and he experienced no pain symptoms. Further, Liam's parents had normally functioning digestive tracts, and his brother, who was presumably being offered the same food, was chubby.

"Are you worried about getting too heavy?" I asked Liam, thinking about his brother and wondering if Liam was restricting his food intake for emotional or psychological reasons relating to his sibling's weight.

"No, I want to get bigger. But I can't make myself eat any more," he asserted.

So what was Liam eating? That was the next piece of information I needed to get. I asked Liam to keep a food diary, writing down everything he ate for several days. Parents fill out this diary for younger children, but when kids reach the age of twelve or so, the exercise is a very helpful way to engage them and make them more aware of what they put—or don't put—in their mouths. A food diary is revealing, because most children, as well as adults, are not truly conscious of what they eat on a daily basis, or how much or little that might be. As I mentioned earlier, I recommend it as a good first step for nearly any nutritional issue.

It was clear from what Liam wrote down that he was pretty finicky. He didn't eat many fruits and vegetables, relying instead on quick and easy carbohydrates. For example, one day for breakfast, he ate four pieces of white toast with cinnamon sugar, juice, and hot cocoa; another day he had eggs on half a bagel and cocoa. His food consumption petered off through the rest of the day. For lunch he picked at the school lunch offering (which consisted of pizza, pasta, or some other fast-food–type meal), and would then eat a few bites of everything offered at dinner. His mother would lay out a spread of steak or other meat, french fries or pasta, skim milk, salad, and banana bread or dessert. She also gave him a multivitamin supplement because she thought it could not hurt. It was one of the popular "gummy" vitamins, which contained tiny amounts of a handful of nutrients but was noticeably missing a number of important vitamins and minerals.

This was not a perfect diet, but it is fairly typical. In fact, it is close to what my nephew eats, and at fifteen, he is 6 feet tall. There are two differences between Liam and my nephew. First, I have watched my nephew polish off half a tray of homemade pasta and wash it down with a few Mountain Dews. Liam's diet could have contained plenty of calories except that his portions, after breakfast, were tiny.

BIO-INDIVIDUALITY

The second difference is accounted for by the great mystery of bio-individuality, or individual biological differences. Everyone has biological quirks that make them need more of this nutrient than the average person or be more intolerant of that food. Two people can eat exactly the same diet with entirely different consequences: One person can grow and feel terrific, and the other person can have stunted growth and be tired. Something about my nephew and half the other kids in the world may allow them to thrive on a diet that would not support Liam. Is it genes, prenatal nutrition, family environment, a minor unnoticed dietary variant, the number of illnesses he had as an infant? It could literally be any one or all those things (or something else entirely). For all we know, the difference could be that my nephew's Italian grandmother lovingly rolls out by hand most of the pasta he consumes. Or there could be a slight nutrient difference between fresh homemade pasta and the boxed stuff. Maybe Liam just has a touchy gene expression that requires him to be more careful with his diet.

We all know someone who lived to the ripe old age of ninety-six and was healthy as a horse even though he smoked cigars and ate ice cream cones every day. This is not the norm or a model for what most of us need to live long and well. Just because some people seem to survive okay eating marginally does not make this a working plan for everyone. The important question was: What was Liam's unique bio-individual characteristic that was getting in the way of normal appetite and growth?

Even though I suspected that a missing nutrient was the root cause for his small stature, I had to admit that aside from being pint-sized, Liam was otherwise very healthy. One would think malnutrition would cause a large number of noticeable problems, and it can. But malnutrition can also be subtle and mild, visible in only one area. In chapter 9 you will see how essential fatty acid deficiency affects the skin. Perhaps Liam was using what nutrients he had to run the immune system, so he was running short (excuse the pun) in only one area.

His parents, represented by his mother, were not ready to explore individual areas of weak nutrition because they were not satisfied that all medical reasons for his small stature had been ruled out. The offhand way in which Liam had been consigned to the fifth percentile continued to bother them. I sensed we would not make much more progress with this family until the growth hormone question had been put to rest.

Thinking I know the answer to a problem and getting a family to accept my analysis and go along with the accompanying plan to fix it are two completely different things. Therefore, I decided to take a two-pronged approach, leading with a plan to settle the growth hormone question, followed closely by a nutrition strategy to close the gap between what Liam was eating and what he needed to grow.

I sent Liam to see another endocrinologist for a more thorough assessment of his growth hormone status even though I did not think growth hormone was a problem. Wendy believed science should have the answer to her son's issue and was not convinced Liam had been fully evaluated, despite the number of doctors she had consulted. I wanted her to feel like someone was listening and to close the growth hormone discussion once and for all. Besides, malnutrition can cause growth hormone deficiency, and maybe Liam's low level of food consumption over a long period of time had caused his growth hormone levels to fall. Growth hormone would be prescribed only if he absolutely needed it, because the drug is injected daily and is expensive. If Liam did need the hormone, using it along with the nutrition program I was planning would speed up his improvement. Both he and his parents needed reassurance from a physician they trusted. I knew just the doctor.

ALL ABOUT GROWTH HORMONE TESTING

I sent Liam to Dr. John J. Merendino Jr., a Maryland-based endocrinologist and coauthor of *The New York Times* bestselling book *The Best*

Life Guide to Managing Diabetes and Pre-Diabetes. He listened carefully to Liam's family's worries and agreed that, given Liam's small stature, it was a good idea for him to be tested to make sure he did not have a growth hormone deficiency. According to Dr. Merendino, growth hormone (GH) deficiency can be accurately confirmed only by using a GH stimulation test. But before we get into that, a few words on how growth hormone works.

GH is made in the pituitary gland and needed for proper growth and wound repair. Despite its name, GH does not directly make a child grow. Instead, it indirectly causes growth by traveling to the liver and stimulating it to excrete insulinlike growth factor-1 (IGF-1). IGF-1 is the actual substance that communicates the growth message to the bones and other tissues. So when doctors test for growth hormone problems in children with stunted growth, they screen the blood for IGF-1, not growth hormone levels.

"IGF-1 is always measured in kids where you are worried about a growth hormone deficiency," Dr. Merendino explained. Then he cautioned that because IGF-1 is a screening test and not precise, the best, most thorough way to find out if there is in fact a deficiency involves a GH challenge. Unfortunately, the GH challenge test requires close medical supervision and a half day at the hospital.

After fasting for ten to twelve hours, Liam had a blood sample drawn. Next, he was given an intravenous solution, which can be either clonidine or arginine. Liam got arginine. Blood samples were drawn at timed intervals, and Liam's GH levels were tested each time. The goal was to see if the arginine properly stimulated his pituitary gland to produce sufficient GH. When he analyzed the results of Liam's test, Dr. Merendino pronounced his growth hormone levels perfect.

As a quick aside, an older, more dangerous version of the challenge test uses insulin as the growth hormone stimulant, but Dr. Merendino recommends avoiding this protocol. One child I saw who needed this test lived in a city where the children's hospital still used insulin. The endocrinologist tried to dissuade the parents from doing the test because it was "dangerous." However, the hospital policy was to use insulin; the parents felt they had no choice if they wanted the information about their child's growth hormone levels. They persisted despite the risks; the child flunked the test, and the doctor confirmed that growth hormone was needed.

WORKING WITH LIAM

The thorough growth hormone evaluation calmed down Liam's parents a lot, and they were now fully committed to other approaches. In the meantime, they had been tentatively embarking on the second prong of my plan, which was closing the nutrient gap between what Liam felt he could eat and what we needed him to eat to grow. In this country, most of us assume that malnutrition occurs only among the poor who go to bed hungry, eat only one meal a day, and otherwise don't have access

SUPER-SMELLERS AND SUPER-TASTERS ARE OFTEN LOW IN ZINC

Many picky eaters complain that food "smells bad" or "tastes funny"—these are the excuses they use for rejecting your famous chicken dish or a different brand of yogurt. Some children will not even sit at the table with the rest of the family because of the allegedly offensive dinner smells.

One popular view of this phenomenon is that the children are super-tasters, equivalent in talent to the sommelier at an expensive French restaurant. Not true. All of the picky-eating "super-tasters" I have taste-tested need visual or contextual cues to accurately identify a taste. They need to see the slight change in color of their preferred yogurt or feel the texture of the pea in the casserole to trigger their aversion.

That is not to say that food does not actually smell or taste "off" to them. The problem is their taste and smell experience is out of sync. We do not know exactly what they are tasting or smelling, but a ripe banana may taste not sweet but sour to them, for example. Or onions being sautéed smell like vomit rather than the beginnings of a delicious dinner. These super-sensitive tasters/smellers are usually picky eaters with a mild zinc deficiency. With a zinc supplement, the excessive numbers of foods with "off" smells and yucky flavors are reduced to a normal level. Like everyone, they still prefer some smells and flavors and avoid others, so not liking onions is not necessarily a sign of zinc deficiency.

to regular meals. But in fact, even children in developed countries who have plenty of choices for how to get calories often self-select foods without enough other nutrients.

One of the unexpected symptoms that can develop when children are not eating well is that they stop feeling hungry—especially when the missing nutrient is zinc. You would think they would be hungrier because their body would want to locate and consume the missing nutrient. And in fact, some children *are* hungrier and overeat. But some lose interest in food. The reactions are individual.

Liam was from a comfortable family, but his diet was still lacking in nutrition. The very popular white diet (high in pasta, milk, bread; low in fruits and vegetables and in meat) contains next to no zinc, an essential mineral for growth. I suspected he was malnourished in this specific nutrient. Liam was surviving on "white" carbohydrates and milk products, both of which lack zinc. Zinc is found in meat, nuts, and seeds. Liam ate meat but not enough to get the amount of zinc he needed. As mentioned before, my theory was that Liam had a mild nutrient deficiency,

TWO WAYS TO TEST FOR ZINC

There are a couple of simple ways to screen for zinc deficiency. The first is a blood test. Your doctor will have to write a prescription for serum zinc levels, because blood tests require a doctor's order. Zinc levels are not part of a regular blood-screening panel, so the doctor must specifically request it. Even children who are veterans of many blood tests rarely come to my office having been screened for zinc deficiency unless they have seen a nutritionally oriented physician. Liam, for example, had not been tested, despite his numerous consultations with specialists.

I rarely ask parents to get their kids a blood test for zinc unless they need to have other blood work done anyway. Kids hate to be poked, and they are often already anxious about the dietary changes we are making in their lives. If I mention a blood test in their presence, the conversation stops, any spirit of cooperation goes out the window, and everything has to be renegotiated.

Instead, I use a screening taste test. The screening test identifies the more subtle deficiency symptoms affecting taste. I test their taste acuity using a zinc sulfate compound. There are a few versions

probably zinc, which was suppressing his appetite. He may have had other micronutrient deficiencies such as magnesium and chromium, because his white diet is low in a number of vitamins and minerals, but those nutrients do not directly affect growth.

In the wild, an animal that doesn't eat and thrive when food is available is eaten by predators. We are still animals (some of us more than others). Liam was surviving, but was starting to get "eaten" on the basketball court and in social areas. For example, his tiny stature was not earning him points with girls. Because hunger is a basic human drive, not being hungry is a huge red flag that something is amiss. Why would a child's survival instincts not be working?

Liam was old enough for me to speak frankly about his size. If a child is old enough—generally at least eleven or twelve—appealing to him or her directly can be very effective. The key is talking to the child as an equal partner in health decisions, rather than as a teacher or boss. Liam made it clear to me that he wished he were bigger and stronger so he could participate in more sports at school. I explained that his body

---

commercially available, such as Zinc Tally (Metagenics) and Zinc Assay (Premier Research Labs). Follow the directions on the bottles, because the amount the child needs to consume for the test may differ. The liquid is clear and has no smell, so there are no clues about how it should taste. I tell the child we are going to play a game and they have to tell me what this mystery drink is. "It is something you know," I hint, "but I am going to try to fool you, so it may be water."

The solution has a strong, disgusting flavor reminiscent of old eggs (caused by the sulfur–part of the sulfate–compound), and if the child can taste it, he makes a face and complains. (Because of this possibility, I always have a glass of water sitting next to the glass with the zinc sulfate, so the child can wash away the flavor.) But for kids who have a zinc deficiency, the zinc sulfate solution has a nondistinct taste or no taste at all. Yes, I am playing a little trick when I claim the solution is something they're familiar with, but because I test only children I am fairly sure are low in zinc, it's rare for a child to have to gulp down the second glass of water to dilute the bad taste. Zinc testing solutions can be bought online if you want to test your family.

needed more nutrients to grow. I also explained that he needed to start introducing new foods—not only to expand the types of foods he was currently eating but to get accustomed to eating and trying new or unfamiliar foods. I didn't think a couple of broccoli spears would make him start to grow immediately, but this approach broadens the adolescent's experience with eating. I was reaching beyond just gaining inches and into enjoying food and setting up healthy eating for life. Liam was out of touch with his appetite, and his diet was monotonous. Over the course of a few months, he ended up finding several new foods he liked, including some vegetables.

It's important for parents to keep in mind that encouraging a child who isn't hungry to eat doesn't help much. If your child has little appetite, telling him to eat doesn't make sense to him. He will perhaps eat a few more bites than he would on his own, but not enough to close a growth gap. One mother reported that if she pressured him, her fifteen-year-old son, who was 5 feet 9 inches but weighed only 103 pounds, would eat a whopping five bites of chicken at dinner. "He wants to go away on weekend school events," she lamented, "but if I am not there pushing him to eat all day, he would starve." Like Liam, this child's appetite is not normal, and a parent constantly cajoling him was helping only minimally.

I returned to my theory that Liam was low in zinc, knowing that zinc is the most effective nutrient for normalizing appetite. The key word is *normalize.* Zinc will not cause people to overeat. So first, I gave Liam a zinc test (see page 112), which he failed with flying colors, indicating that he was indeed low in zinc. I then gave him a comprehensive multivitamin/mineral plus an additional supplement containing 20 milligrams more of zinc. The zinc would improve his urge to eat while helping his smell and taste acuity.

I also encouraged him to eat two to three servings of fruits and vegetables per day to improve the quality of his diet. He established this habit over several months. Fruits and vegetables were not going to add significant calories, but over the long run, a broader diet would serve his health better. Besides, he was not going to get more flexible as the teenage years progressed, so there was no time like the present to encourage new food experiences.

At first, it was a chore for him to eat his carrots, but we talked about what might be good to try, starting with apples, oranges, and peas. Each time we met, we agreed on two or three more foods to try. Gradually, he was not only growing but eating a broader diet. Although zinc can perk up the appetite, kids will often just eat more of the same boring foods they were eating before. My goal was quantity and quality.

You are probably wondering why Liam would add vegetables to his diet for me (a stranger) and not his mother or father. Oh, how I wish I could claim that the reason is my uncommon brilliance, but alas the explanation is more prosaic. No parent likes to hear this, but kids are more often willing to try harder for strangers

The Zinc List

Improve your child's zinc status by including these zinc-rich foods in his diet:

FOOD	MILLIGRAMS OF ZINC PER SERVING
beef (3 oz.)	8.9
king crab (3 oz.)	6.5
pork shoulder (3 oz.)	4.2
poultry (chicken leg)	2.7
baked beans (½ cup)	1.7
cashews (1 oz.)	1.6
pumpkin seeds (⅔ oz.)	1.3
chickpeas (½ cup)	1.3

Foods that contain less than 1 mg of zinc per serving (or weak sources of zinc): milk, white meat chicken, peanut butter, cheese, oatmeal.

and authority figures who are not their parents. Not always, but surprisingly often. (Ask any teacher, coach, or therapist.) Liam knew his mother would still love him even if he never touched a vegetable, so when the going got tough, he could blow off the broccoli. He was not sure what I would think about him, and he wanted to be seen as competent.

Find professionals with whom you can talk and who share your values.

Nobody wants to have their deepest concerns cavalierly dismissed by being told not to worry. Your health care provider should respect your concerns enough to at least address them with thoughtfulness. Studies in the art of persuasion show that people are much more likely to go along with an idea if an explanation is given.

A number of years ago, I set a very high standard for the health care professionals I see and send my clients to: I have to like them. They don't have to be my best friend, but I want to look forward to, not dread, a visit with them. How much healing can take place if you are sitting in the waiting room with a knot in your stomach?

When I began working with Liam in April, he weighed seventy pounds; by July he weighed seventy-five pounds; by August he weighed seventy-seven pounds. He had also grown several inches! By the end of the year he weighed seventy-nine pounds and had grown five and a half inches. Taking his supplements with extra zinc had picked up his appetite, so he started feeling hungry and ate more. His palate also became more adventurous because he discovered new foods he liked. Now he could find something to eat when he went out rather than eating only a few bites if one his favorite limited foods were not available. And he gained the necessary weight to grow. These were remarkable results using easy-to-find, safe, over-the-counter remedies and small dietary changes.

WHY ZINC IS IMPORTANT

The first recognized cases of zinc deficiency were reported in 1963, when stunted growth and delayed sexual maturation in a group of Egyptian boys were linked to diets poor in zinc. The boys' growth and development improved with zinc supplements, and these findings were duplicated in children all over the world. Since then, we have learned more about the complex relationship between growth hormone (GH), insulinlike growth factor-1 (IGF-1), and this essential trace mineral. Bottom line: If your levels of zinc are low enough, you won't grow, and low zinc intake is surprisingly common in children who are not growing to their genetic potential. It's interesting to note as well that giving zinc to children who also have a clear growth hormone deficiency has shown to increase their stature more than taking GH alone. But the benefits do not stop at growth. Zinc is also critical for taste and smell acuity, proper wound healing, and immune function. Deficiency symptoms include hair loss (also known as alopecia), skin lesions and dermatitis, developmental delays, and altered behavior. According to Ananda Prasad—aka Dr. Zinc, because he was the first researcher to report cases of zinc deficiency—zinc is involved in more than three hundred enzyme and hormone pathways.

Despite its importance, dietary surveys continue to find that many people, even in America, are mildly deficient in zinc. Zinc is easily available in developed countries, where the average grocery store is overflowing with meat and nuts (see "The Zinc List" on page 115 for foods that are good sources of zinc). Unfortunately, many children choose not to eat much from the meat and nut departments, preferring the cereal (most kid cereal does not include "added" zinc) and pasta aisles. Absorption problems can also affect zinc status. An amazing number of substances lurking around interfere with zinc absorption. Many medications, such as those prescribed for reflux, prevent zinc uptake. Environmental toxins such as mercury and lead literally take zinc out of the body. Between low intake and absorption troubles, zinc is an at-risk nutrient.

Should You Be Concerned About Your Child's Growth?

Having a short child is not necessarily cause for concern. At the same time, the blithe advice to "wait and see" doesn't always properly address the symptoms and situation. Answering the following questions can help you determine if your child has a hormonal growth issue that requires further medical or nutritional investigation.

☐ Is your child in the fifth percentile or lower for weight or height according to a standard growth chart?

☐ Is your child's growth trend going down dramatically? For example, has he dropped more than 20 percent on the growth chart and ended up in the tenth percentile or below?

☐ Does your child rarely seem to be hungry? Or, can you easily stay on a food budget with a male preteen or teenager in the house? If you can, be very suspicious. Girls' appetites should increase, too, but not as dramatically.

☐ Is your child a very picky eater?

☐ Does your child complain frequently that food smells or tastes "funny"?

☐ Does your underweight child get full after a few bites (not counting dessert)?

☐ Has a bone-age test found that your small child's bone age is close to her chronological age?

If you answered yes to two or more of these questions, consider these next steps.

What to Do

1. Make an appointment to talk to your doctor only about your child's weight and height. Don't bring up any other health concerns until you receive full answers to your questions. If you go to the doctor with a multipoint agenda, she will address the issue she is most concerned about or knows the most about, and that may not be your child's size.

2. Make a plan with your doctor that you are comfortable with. If your child is ten or younger and she suggests watching and waiting, nail down a time frame and a specific set of tests you will do at that time or the specialist you will see if growth does not improve. A good noninvasive test to request is bone aging. If your child is six but has a bone age of

four, then his size and weight may be average for his bone age. This means your child's body thinks he is four and is growing accordingly. In general, you want the bone age to be behind his chronological age in a small child.

3. If the child is eleven or older, do not agree to watch and wait but ask for a referral to an endocrinologist. Why? Because if your child is a candidate for growth hormone therapy and the child goes into puberty, it is too late. GH works only before puberty, and the child needs time to grow.

4. Consider a zinc supplement for your child. A general recommendation to address growth issues would be 20 milligrams for children ages three to five and 30 milligrams for children ages six years and older, but talk to a knowledgeable medical professional if you have specific questions about your child.

5. If you are uncomfortable with what you are hearing, get another opinion or two. One of the families in my practice saw four endocrinologists before they found one who listened and properly diagnosed their son's growth problem.

6. If your child's appetite does not pick up, find a good nutritionist to help balance his diet and add appropriate nutritional supplements.

CHAPTER 8

The Little Colon That Couldn't

I N MY JOB, PARENTS TALK TO ME FREQUENTLY about their children's bowel movements or lack thereof. This topic comes with the territory, and I am quite used to it by now. Parents are relieved to be able to share the details of their concerns. "Getting her to poop is such a big deal; is that normal?" one mother shared with me. Another exasperated mother confessed, "I feel like I'm still toilet-training, trying to figure out how to make my six-year-old go to the bathroom regularly." "He only goes every three days, and then there is so much, it clogs up the toilet," another woman admitted with embarrassment. "Where does he keep it all?"

I hear versions of these comments all too often. We all know how important it is for our body's excretory system to work properly, and this is especially true of children's. A youngster who is having a bowel movement only every three days, four days, or once a week cannot be comfortable. Nor can it be healthy to keep all those waste products inside. A clogged-up colon at any age can turn an otherwise happy day into a trial.

CONSTIPATION IS COMMON

A lot of kids have constipation, but parents often don't recognize it as such. For instance, a child who has a bowel movement (BM) every three days is constipated, even if the movement is soft. "But the doctor says a BM every three days or even once a week is normal," parents report. Common, yes; normal, no. Would you leave the remains of your dinner on your kitchen table for three days? No, it would get smelly and is unsanitary. Leaving the remains of breakfast, lunch, and dinner inside you for days causes the same problem. Rotting food acted on by bacteria living along the gut lining needs to be excreted before it starts generating toxins such as putrescine and cadaverine.

Ever wonder why intestinal gas smells? Putrescine is the same clear, malodorous fume that is emitted from rotting corpses, which is where it was first identified. Cadaverine is a close relative, as you can guess from its name. And they not only smell bad but react with other common chemicals in the body and form carcinogens. Some is expelled and some is absorbed. Your ten-year-old is correct: Gas is gross. Best to move the food along and maintain the right bacteria balance to reduce the production of untoward by-products.

Some smells associated with BMs are the result of normal processing. How much smell and the composition and toxicity of the chemicals creating the odor depend on the types of organisms living in the gut, the diet, and how long the food leftovers are dallying there. The most logical excretion pattern would be a BM for every meal: new food in, old food out. Most of us have trained our bodies to store up our meal remains for at least a day, but this is a social and practical decision, not necessarily the most desirable biologically. Getting rid of refuse as soon as it is finished processing makes the most sense biologically, and that is exactly what most animals and babies do.

We are civilized beings, and most of us seem to have settled on the made-up schedule of three meals a day and eliminating once a day. You can eat more or less often or go to the bathroom more often, but I believe that optimally, you should get rid of the remains of your meals at least

THE MANY FACES OF FIBER

Fiber is simply the part of grains, fruits, and vegetables that your body cannot absorb. There is no fiber in dairy products or meats. Fiber literally goes in one end of the body and out the other. However, its magical power is that while passing through the colon, bacteria act on fiber to produce substances needed to repair the gut lining and stimulate bowel function. The gut lining needs to be repaired frequently, because it is in continuous use and the cells are constantly being rubbed off.

The different types of fibers fall into two categories: soluble or insoluble. Soluble fiber dissolves in water and insoluble does not. Soluble fiber works in the intestine by absorbing water into the stool, but it also conveniently sops up extra cholesterol in your intestines. This is why oatmeal manufacturers advertise its ability to lower cholesterol. All that water absorption has the added benefit of helping you feel full. This is why you can eat one apple, which contains soluble fiber, and feel full, but drink four to six apples' worth of juice without feeling full.

Insoluble fiber actually absorbs a little bit of water, too, but is mostly valued for its ability to bulk up the stool and push it through. Broccoli and bran are loaded with insoluble fiber. However, most whole grains, legumes, fruits, and vegetables have a combination of soluble and insoluble fiber. The Institute of Medicine recommends 14 grams of fiber for every 1,000 calories of food. That works out to about 19 grams a day for kids ages one to three, 25 grams for children ages four to eight, and about 30 grams or so starting at age nine.

once per day. If you go less often without discomfort, most medical professionals do not consider the problem to be constipation; however, I consider this situation suboptimal.

In children, constipation is usually caused by either too little fiber in the diet or withholding. A diet high in refined flour and cheese and/or low in fruits and vegetables (the "white" diet) is the usual culprit. This meal plan is missing fiber, whose sole job is to create a bulky structure for eliminating undigested food. The fastest correction is adding several servings of fruits and vegetables per day to the child's diet, which is also in the best interest of her general health. (See "FFFF—Fun Fiber for Fussy Feeders," on page 131, for some kid-friendly fiber suggestions.)

A second, common cause of constipation is withholding. Toddlers begin to connect the uncomfortable pressure down there with pooping, usually during the process of toilet training. The ability to tie an event to a consequence starts to happen developmentally around the time most little ones are being potty trained. "I don't like this feeling associated with sitting on that strange chair," their baby minds reason. "Maybe I can control my muscles enough to stop it." And thus the withholding begins. According to Dr. Celia Padron, a New Jersey–based pediatric gastroenterologist, it can take just one uncomfortable bowel movement for toddlers to commence withholding. When the stools finally do force their way out, it is even more painful than before, so the toddler starts to exert even more resistance. The good news is that with time and experience and enough fiber and fluid to keep the BMs soft and comfortable to pass, most toddlers overcome withholding.

However, not all cases of constipation are so cut and dried.

SARAH: AN ALL-TOO-COMMON TALE

Three-year-old Sarah was brought to see me by her mother, Claire, who explained that Sarah frequently went five or six days without having a bowel movement. The first few days after elimination were pleasant, but by day four, life revolved around the next BM. Sarah wandered around aimlessly, short-tempered and miserable. I learned that even at fifteen months old, Sarah had difficulty going to the bathroom, and her pediatrician treated the constipation with a common hyperosmotic laxative, which works by retaining water in the colon so the stool can become softer. (See "Meet the Laxative Drugs" on page 128.)

Now almost two years later, despite her continued use of the laxative, Sarah was still having trouble with constipation. In fact, some weeks she was pooping only once, and during better weeks every three or four days. And oh, how they prayed for the good weeks. The days leading up to bowel movement day were increasingly disrupted as Sarah grew more and more irritable. All life revolved around her finally going to the bathroom. Things would move, and everyone would heave a huge sigh of relief.

I asked about Sarah's diet and learned that, like many kids, she was a picky eater, eating few fruits and vegetables and lots of bagels, yogurt, and cheese. A lot of dairy, I thought to myself.

"Have you tried adding more fiber?" I inquired. Claire responded that of course they had tried increasing Sarah's fiber, but that she stopped because the constipation actually got worse during those periods. She had tried several times to force Sarah to eat more fruit and even added bran to her yogurt, but instead of softer, more frequent movements, Sarah went less and was more uncomfortable.

As I continued to delve into Sarah's history, I learned that she had been constipated since birth, even though Claire had nursed her. This was unexpected, because breast milk should not be constipating, making this an important clue.

"Since birth?" I repeated, to be sure. If not from day one, the constipation had certainly started shortly thereafter.

Claire also revealed that since birth, Sarah had had eczema that came and went, although this was of less concern than the bowel issues.

Let's review what we've learned about Sarah so far. Remember, to be a nutrition detective, start with the bones of a stripped-down story. The possible clues so far are as follows:

- chronic constipation
- eczema
- timing: both began before three months of age
- fiber made the constipation worse

Extensive research over the last several decades has linked chronic constipation in children to an intolerance to cow's milk. According to *Pediatrics*, the official journal of the American Pediatric Association, "prudence may suggest that a trial of dietary elimination of cow's milk be undertaken for recalcitrant constipation unresponsive to other therapies." There is also clinical research connecting eczema in children with food sensitivity, usually to some combination of dairy, eggs, and tomatoes. *Some combination* means any one of these items or any combination of the three. Dairy protein (casein) is one of the most reactive substances in the diet, so it comes up as an irritant over and over.

The only glitch in this theory is that Sarah's constipation started with breast-feeding. Clearly she was not eating a cheese burrito at three months of age, so how was she getting cow's milk protein? The answer was through the breast milk. Like most conscientious new mothers, Claire was likely following recommendations for breast-feeding, which usually contain the advice to eat plenty of dairy products for calcium. The casein protein in the cow's milk products Claire was eating can find its way into mother's milk and start the reaction process. I decided to ask Claire about her milk product consumption while she was nursing.

"I followed the advice of the lactation consultant at the hospital," Claire said. "I don't like milk very much, but I ate plenty of yogurt and cheese."

So far, three of our symptom clues can be explained by dairy intolerance. That is about as good a pattern as a detective is likely to find. I went with my theory that removing the dairy products from Sarah's diet would probably help the constipation and eczema, but I also knew that I had to address the additional problem of dependency on laxatives.

First things first: Remove the irritants. I suggested to Claire that we remove dairy products from Sarah's diet. Given how picky Sarah was about food, understandably Claire was not thrilled about taking out a mainstay of Sarah's diet, but desperation is the mother of determination, so she agreed to try. I explained that when irritants are removed, often children are more comfortable and naturally expand their eating preferences.

For extra digestive support, I recommended the addition of probiotics, health-enhancing microorganisms such as those found in yogurt that are being used with children more and more often. Remember how the balance of good bacteria is one of the factors that determine how stinky the stool is? I wanted to tip that balance toward cleaner, more efficient elimination by adding the right bugs.

There are excellent studies done with children suggesting that probiotics may help reduce diarrhea and allergies, and help irritable bowel syndrome, Crohn's disease, infections, and constipation. Although helping this number of conditions is impressive, probiotics have the additional benefit of being safe and nontoxic. Occasionally, they will cause some gas and bloat, so I always have parents start with a quarter or half of the intended dose and work up slowly over one to two weeks. I put Sarah on a product that contained about ten billion bugs. It contained a number

How to Select a Good Probiotic

Probiotics are live microorganisms, usually but not always bacteria. By consuming them, you can boost your own population of desirable bugs and possibly protect yourself against disease-causing microbes, commonly referred to as germs. There are dozens of strains of "good" bacteria that may benefit your health. They have long, complicated names such as *Lactobacillus acidophilus*, *Bifidobacterium lactis*, and even *Streptococcus thermophilus* (which sounds bad but is actually good for you). Small amounts are present in foods such as yogurt, miso, and other fermented juices or drinks, but to get their therapeutic effects you may have to consume larger amounts, which are available in capsules and powder.

Different companies market a specific species or a proprietary blend of bugs. The potency is usually listed as an estimated number of live bacteria (such as ten billion) or as colony-forming units. Because the organisms are heat-sensitive, the product should be sold from the refrigerator unless it is stabilized. Bug numbers deteriorate significantly with time, heat, and moisture, not to mention the digestive process, so the more you can do to keep the bugs alive by storing them in a cool, dry environment, the better. Excellent products guarantee potency through a posted expiration date. Good luck proving the organisms are dead or alive by that date, but it is still nice to see.

If you are concerned about the quality of a particular product, ConsumerLab (www.consumerlab.com), a for-profit laboratory, tests the potency of many supplements, including probiotics, to see if their contents match what is on the label. For a fee, you can check out the quality of a number of popular products. Although 93 percent of the probiotics tested in one report did not contain the number of live organisms listed on the bottle, most still had enough live good bugs to be potentially beneficial.

Look for a product that contains more than a billion bugs. Ten billion or more is even better. By comparison, a tub of yogurt may contain a few of different species of good bacteria and required refrigeration. (For more information, see "How to Select a Good Probiotic" below.)

The first several days without dairy were dicey when it came to eating. Claire frequently offered her the few nondairy items on her menu, such as pasta and fruit, and Sarah ate them but repeatedly asked for cheese. Claire was tempted to give her just a little because Sarah looked so forlorn, but she held firm and suggested other choices. By the end of the first week, Sarah started picking items off Claire's or her sister's plate

hundred million good bacteria and almost never lists which strain is used in production. Some supplements also contain prebiotics, which are selective food or fertilizers for the probiotics. Good bacteria need food to grow, just like children. Fructooligosaccharrides and inulin are the most common prebiotics. The trend in prescribing probiotics has moved toward using products with higher numbers of bacteria rather than supplements containing a combination of probiotics and prebiotics. However, both types of supplements can help. Direct questions about your individual situation to a knowledgeable health care provider.

Research on probiotics almost alwawys focuses on a specific strain of a microbe species. The first word in the name (such as *Lactobacillus*) is the genus. It may be abbreviated to a letter (*L.*). The species is the second name (such as *rhamnosus*). The strain is the last part of the name (such as *GG*). Put it together and you have *L. rhamnosus GG*. Different strains have different effects, so those who are research-minded

may want to look up the data on their condition of most concern (for Sarah it would be constipation) and pick a product containing a strain that has been shown to help that problem. Two strains that have been studied specifically for constipation are *Bifidobacterium lactis* and *Lactobacillus casei Shirota*, but many people find that any probiotic helps constipation.

I tend to be less precise. Generally, children respond well to a variety of products readily available at the health food store. And just as rotating crops helps keep soil healthy, rotating probiotics can maximize exposure to a larger number of potentially helpful microorganisms. If your child doesn't yet swallow pills, you will have to open the capsules or take a dose of a powder version and mix it in applesauce, juice, or other food that is cool or at room temperature. Remember, these bugs cannot withstand much heat. The only products I rarely recommend are chewable probiotics. The number of live organisms in them tends to be too small for therapeutic purposes.

and putting them in her mouth. She discovered she liked fish with tartar sauce. Perhaps the creamy sauce reminded her of milk.

Within a few weeks, Sarah was pooping more regularly. She was still taking the laxative, but she was more comfortable and, as hoped, eating a wider variety of foods. Because she hadn't pushed out a regular bowel movement for more than a year and a half, owing to the early introduction of laxatives, it would take several months for her bowel muscles to get used to performing peristalsis on their own. Peristalsis is the wave-like, coordinated muscle contractions that move food along the digestive tract toward the rectum.

After a few months passed and Sarah was pooping easily and daily, Claire tried to reduce the laxative slowly, but with any reduction in the medicine, Sarah immediately stopped having daily bowel movements.

Meet the Laxative Drugs

A laxative is a substance that induces a bowel movement. The best way to avoid laxatives is to increase the intake of fibers found in vegetables, fruits, and whole grains. Many of us are not eating enough of these foods, as evidenced by the $725 million a year Americans spend on over-the-counter laxatives. Some fiber products dissolve easily into fluids like juice and are well tolerated by children. All the other laxatives described are available in a kid-friendly liquid or chewable form.

BULK-FORMING AGENT, OR FIBER IN A CAN. These are the safest and gentlest types of laxative because they are similar to substances naturally found in food. A diet full of whole grains, legumes, fruits, and vegetables does not need to be supplemented with fiber. For those not eating a perfect diet, fiber can be purchased in a can and added. These products are powdery or grainy and dissolve in fluid. They increase the size of the stool because fiber is not digested and stays in the digestive tract. A stool has to have a little size (bulk) so it can be pushed along and eventually out. There has to be enough bulk in a stool so the pressure receptors in the rectum know there is something there to push out. Commercial examples of this type of laxative are Benefiber and Metamucil.

STOOL SOFTENERS OR SURFACTANTS pull fat and water into the stool, making it softer, bulkier, and easier to push along, but the body adapts to them quickly, so they are good only for occasional use. The most common brand is Colace.

"The doctor says it is no big deal to just keep her on the medicine, since she is finally comfortable and it is not habit-forming," Claire reported.

Although these were valid arguments, I encouraged Claire to take Sarah to the next level of bowel health.

People are not robbing convenience stores for hyperosmotic laxatives, and they are not technically addictive or adaptive. But their long-term use can be problematic nonetheless. Many children, like Sarah, cannot seem to function without them. I could fill a small bowel-rehab center just with the kids who have walked through my door with this issue. For example, Armand, at age five, had been on a similar laxative since he was six months old and had never had an unassisted bowel movement. Even small reductions in the laxative dosage resulted in

---

LUBRICANTS work like WD-40 in the gut, helping the stool slip along. Most of the commercial lubricants are based in mineral oil. I do not like mineral oil because it is a petroleum-based product and may form an indigestible film that could reduce the absorption of fat-soluble vitamins and some minerals. It is not used much anymore, thank goodness, but I always suggest other alternatives when I run into someone still taking it.

STIMULANTS, the most aggressive and dangerous of the laxatives, work on the intestinal lining to induce peristalsis. These laxatives can cause a "cathartic effect" (or a violent emptying episode) and are the most associated with laxative abuse and long-term problems. Do not give these to children without doctor supervision. Common stimulant laxatives include Ex-Lax and Dulcolax.

HYDRATING AGENTS are the most commonly prescribed laxatives for constipation in children. There are two types: saline (salt-based) and hyperosmotic. The salts, such as milk of magnesia or Epsom salt, simply retain water in the intestine. Hyperosmotic agents are made up of other substances, such as lactulose and polyethylene glycol, that retain water in the colon. The reason extra water in the colon may be useful is that a stool sitting for too long can get too dry and hard to push along. The main purpose of the large intestine is to reabsorb water into the body. A long-standing stool (as in constipation) keeps having more and more water removed until it is a shriveled-up, smelly prune. How is that for an image? Some common brand names are GlycoLax, CoLyte, and MiraLAX.

immediate constipation. Harry, at age four, was taking an adult-size dose of an osmotic laxative along with an adult-size dose of a stimulant laxative to have regular BMs. This is just the tip of the iceberg.

WHEN FIBER GOES WRONG

If osmotic laxatives are not addicting, why do so many children have trouble getting off them? One clue I have noticed is that these same children tend to get more constipated if extra fiber is added to their diets. As mentioned before, constipation is typically treated by increasing fiber (found in fruits, vegetables, and whole grains). But when a child has low muscle tone, too much fiber actually makes things worse.

Hypotonia is the medical term used to describe muscles with a floppy, toneless quality, and although these muscles can also be weak, they are not necessarily so. It can be hard to see low muscle tone, especially in the trunk and abdominal area, but some telltale signs are frequent slumping, low stamina, and poor posture. A protruding belly in an otherwise normal-weight child is also a symptom.

> A dramatic increase in fiber intake when a child has low muscle tone is equivalent to trying to help a person who never goes to the gym by asking her to lift extra weight.

Children can have generalized low muscle tone or just be hypotonic in a specific area or areas of the body. But low muscle tone in the trunk and lower abdomen means they can have trouble pushing out bowel movements. Imagine going to the gym when you are out of shape and having trouble lifting the weights. Would adding extra weight help? Of course not. A dramatic increase in fiber intake when a child has low muscle tone is equivalent to trying to help a person who never goes to the gym by asking her to lift extra weight. A child needs well-developed internal muscles for easy peristalsis just like you need well-developed external muscles to lift heavy weights. If the muscles are not strong enough, you need another

FFFF — FUN FIBER FOR FUSSY FEEDERS

Here are some of the more kid-friendly high-fiber foods and their fiber contents:

- baked beans in sauce (½ cup), 8 grams
- whole-wheat egg noodles (1 cup cooked), 5.7 grams
- apple (medium), 4 grams
- pear (medium), 4 grams
- sweet-potato fries (about 1 cup), 4 grams
- whole-wheat English muffin, 3.7 grams
- raisin bran (½ cup), 3.7 grams (Note: Fiber amount may vary by brand. Check label.)
- carrots (½ cup cooked), 3.4 grams
- strawberries (1 cup), 3 grams
- watermelon (1 thick slice), 2.8 grams
- orange (large), 2.4 grams
- baby carrots (raw, 2 oz.), 2 grams
- peanut butter without stabilizers or extra oil (1 tablespoon), 1.5 grams
- popcorn (1 cup), 1 gram
- raisins (1 tablespoon), 1 gram

For extremely finicky eaters, you can mix one to two tablespoons of prune juice into milk, yogurt, or other juice. They usually do not notice it is there. Pancakes can be made with a heaping tablespoon of bran or ground flaxseeds added to the batter. You can also buy juice with added fiber online. Regular commercial juice does not contain fiber because it is filtered and clarified to remove the pulp and any other particles that might be fibrous. Unfiltered juice or juice with pulp may contain some fiber.

---

strategy, gradually toning and strengthening the muscles by slowly increasing the load.

Serious hypotonia is part of the profile of a number of conditions such as muscular dystrophy, genetic syndromes such as Down syndrome, and mitochondria disorders. Infants born prematurely can also have tone issues. Consequently, constipation frequently accompanies physical developmental delays. Mild low muscle tone, on the other hand, is generally benign, so it is rarely noticed even though it is relatively common and, to some degree, normal in young children. Symptoms include delays in developing head control, trouble sitting up straight or a preference for lying on the floor, poor stamina, a mouth that hangs open or excessive drooling, and a "Buddha belly."

I suspected Sarah had some mild problems with low trunk tone. Her mother could not confirm any particular symptoms except that she did get tired easily and had lain around a lot while waiting for bowel movements in the past. In my experience, building internal muscles is tricky, but I have found one technique that works consistently well: the addition of a special protein called carnitine. Carnitine is a simple protein made up of the two amino acid building blocks methionine and lysine. Ninety-eight percent of the body's carnitine resides in the muscles. L-carnitine is the supplement form of carnitine that best helps the muscles. Other forms, such as acetyl-L-carnitine, are used more frequently for cognitive enhancement.

Carnitine has a number of functions, such as transporting fats into the mitochondria so they can be burned for energy. Athletes, especially weight lifters, like carnitine because it reportedly increases endurance and lean muscle mass. In fact, if you buy a bottle of carnitine, the label may feature a picture of a buff abdomen or bulging biceps to highlight its valued muscle-building effect. What you will not see is a picture of the pink insides of an intestine, yet for the purposes of constipation, L-carnitine's most relevant function is enhancing the contraction of muscles, specifically those in the bowel.

To help Sarah improve bowel tone, we slowly added liquid L-carnitine to her regimen while reducing the osmotic laxative. This process took several months because her muscles needed time to get exercised and built up. If you add a full corrective dose of L-carnitine immediately, intestinal cramps, nausea, and/or diarrhea are the usual result. L-carnitine is found mostly in meat, but increasing dietary sources does not improve constipation. (As if eating meat would improve constipation!) Why it works when taken as a supplement and not when it is buried in food is a nutrition mystery.

This was our process for Sarah: Claire added 250 milligrams of L-carnitine the first day while leaving the laxative at the regular dose of one capful per day. Usually, the carnitine loosens the stools, allowing the laxative to be reduced slightly. Sarah's stools were looser, so we reduced the laxative by one-fourth and watched the stools over the next week. Sure enough, the addition of the L-carnitine with three-fourths of a capful of laxative kept the bowel movements soft and regular. If the 250 milligrams of carnitine had caused diarrhea, we would have reduced the laxative to half a dose right away.

We let Sarah adjust to the reduced medicine and carnitine for a few weeks and then made

> NUTRITION DETECTIVE PRINCIPLE #8
>
> ## A BM a day keeps the GI specialist away.
>
> Do not accept weekly bowel movements as regular or normal. Every child should poop at least once or twice a day. Period.
>
> It's best to start good bowel habits early, beginning by slowly increasing the fiber in your child's diet.

another move, only this time we reduced the laxative to half a capful the same day we increased the carnitine to 500 milligrams. The adjustment went smoothly, pardon the pun, and all was going well until Sarah got a cold. She did not have a BM one day, and Claire panicked. Relatives were expected in a few days for a visit, and she did not want to go back to the bad old constipation days. We decided to hold at the half dose of laxative and 500 milligrams of carnitine for a month, and Claire tried to keep Sarah's fluids up during her illness. She was back on schedule within a few days, and a month later we marched on.

Sarah's L-carnitine supplement was increased to 750 milligrams and the laxative reduced to a quarter capful. At this point the laxative dose was so low and Sarah was so accustomed to normal bowel movements that after a few weeks, we just skipped the laxatives every other day to see what would happen. Her bowel movements continued to be regular. A month later, she was permanently off laxatives.

If your child has similar issues, discuss the situation with your health care practitioner before reducing prescribed laxatives or adding L-carnitine. L-carnitine is generally prescribed therapeutically at doses of 50 to 100 milligrams per kilogram of body weight. A kilogram equals approximately 2.2 pounds. Take your child's weight in pounds and divide it by 2.2 to get her weight in kilograms. That number (weight in kilograms) times 100 is the most L-carnitine you would want to use.

Does Your Child's Constipation Stem From a Reaction to Milk?

The goal here is to figure out why your child is constipated. The first thing you want to determine is whether your child's constipation could be related to an excessive amount of dairy in his diet, because that is the more stubborn problem. Ask yourself these questions:

- ☐ Is my child's main source of protein cheese, milk, and/or yogurt?

- ☐ Did the constipation start before one year of age? This could suggest that dairy is a culprit, because the main type of protein in the diet before age one for those consuming formula is casein from cow's milk.

- ☐ Is there a history of problems with infant formula?

- ☐ Did my child have adverse reactions to dairy that he seemed to outgrow? This would suggest a history of dairy problems that may need to be revisited.

- ☐ Does my child prefer drinking milk to eating?

- ☐ Has there been blood in the stool? (This is a well-known medical sign of dairy intolerance.)

A yes answer to any of these questions could point to dairy intolerance or excessive dairy consumption.

Is Your Child's Constipation From Too Little Fiber?

- ☐ Does your child eat a mostly white diet?

- ☐ Does he eat two or fewer servings of fruit and vegetables per day?

- ☐ Does your child avoid whole grains?

- ☐ Is the quantity of his stool small?

- ☐ Is the stool hard and dry?

A yes answer to any of these questions means your child could use more fiber in his diet.

What to Do

1. If your child is not having daily bowel movements and is eating a white diet, begin by increasing fiber slowly. Add an extra serving of fruit or vegetables for one week and then add a second. Be consistent.

2. If additional fiber does not help, or makes things worse, consider removing or dramatically reducing the amount of dairy products. Give your child 800 to 1,000 milligrams of calcium in the form of a supplement—half in the morning and half at night.

3. If your child becomes constipated with toilet training, consider putting off toilet training for a few months and trying again. Walking around in a diaper allows the child to use his leg muscles to help the excretion process. Animals poop while they are walking or standing because it is physiologically easier. Pushing from a seated position requires better muscle development and control, which in some children takes more time. Alternatively, you can try making the process easier by placing a stool under your child's feet when he is sitting so his legs are supported and he can push more easily. If a child's feet are dangling, he cannot use his leg muscles to move the bowels.

4. If your child is laxative dependent and removing dairy products and increasing fiber has not helped, talk to your health care practitioner about weaning him off the medicine using L-carnitine, especially if there are signs of low muscle tone in the trunk area.

CHAPTER 9

A Case of Chicken Skin

IGHT-YEAR-OLD ROBERT CAME TO SEE me because his mother, Jenny, was worried about a stubborn rash that had spread over his entire torso. She could not remember exactly when it started because it seemed as if the little bumps had always been there. Looking back she thought his skin had been smooth as a toddler. "Did he have them when he went to preschool?" I prompted.

Jenny hesitated. "I am not sure—maybe," she ventured. "Kindergarten?" I pressed.

He definitely had them by kindergarten, she could confirm, because another child had made a remark about them. So they probably appeared somewhere between ages three and five. The rash looked like small, raised red goose bumps. What were we looking at? I wondered.

I asked her if I could see Robert's rash, and she readily agreed. His torso was rough, bumpy, and dry but not overly irritated. "Could I see the back side of your arms, too?" I asked Robert. No problem—up went the arms. The skin here was similar to that on the trunk, but the bumps were more distinct and looked exactly like plucked chicken skin. In total, Robert had more "alien" than regular skin. Any parent would understand why it bothered Jenny.

But when asked, Robert claimed the rash did not bother him. He felt no irritation or pain. And as long as he had a T-shirt on, the bumps were only barely visible at the edges of his sleeves. His legs were mildly affected but not enough to cause other children to comment. Overall, he seemed well adjusted and happy.

THE MYSTERY OF ROBERT'S BUMPY SKIN

Jenny had already taken Robert to a dermatologist a few years before who had ruled out eczema because there was no itching or particular irritation. At the time, he had labeled the condition keratosis pilaris (KP), a benign skin condition of unknown origin that the rest of us would call chicken skin.

Keratin is the main structural protein in the outer cell membrane of the skin, and when it builds up and becomes rough and dry, the condition is called keratosis. Although nobody would call Robert unsightly (in fact, he was adorable both inside and out), Jenny did not think her otherwise healthy child should have lumpy skin. Consequently, she dutifully applied every cream suggested or prescribed. But no matter what kind of lotion or gel Jenny slathered on or bathed him in, Robert's bumps did not soften or budge. She pronounced the ointments "worthless" and was mighty upset by the time she arrived at my doorstep.

I asked Jenny if she knew whether Robert were allergic to anything, such as fish, shellfish, or environmental agents. Because his trunk and upper arms were the most widely affected areas, I thought perhaps laundry detergent or chemicals in fabric could be bothering him. Jenny was showing herself to be a good detective. She had already suspected that perhaps Robert's bumpy, dry skin was caused by an allergy. She had requested that his doctor run a general blood test, which turned out negative for allergies. The doctor had tested a wide variety of foods, pollen, dust mites, ragweed, trees, molds, and animal dander.

I then asked Jenny if Robert had any other suspicious symptoms. All she came up with was that Robert was often constipated. Hmm, I thought. The constipation could be a clue I could use. One of the functions of the skin is excreting toxins and other substances. (If you have ever been in close quarters with someone who has eaten too much garlic, you have experienced one way volatile substances literally ooze from the pores—in this case the "volatile" part being the smelly sulfur compounds found in garlic.) Constipation suggests some kind of clogging of the digestive system, so I wondered whether some of the waste products that should be excreted through the bowels were backing up behind the skin.

Next I asked Jenny to describe Robert's diet. It became clear very quickly that Robert was a typical picky eater: lots of white, processed foods, such as frozen breakfasts and toaster pastries, very few fresh fruits or vegetables, and lots of ice cream. Specifically he ate French toast sticks for breakfast; turkey bacon, a minimal number of raw vegetables, and toaster pastries for lunch; and maybe some chocolate milk for a snack. Then he'd have a fairly typical dinner (mostly made up of frozen chicken nuggets and maybe frozen french fries) and always a giant bowl of ice cream for dessert.

No wonder he was constipated! Robert's diet contained barely a gram of fiber! And clearly, there was way too much sugar and processed food. My diet diagnosis was immediate: deficient. He did not have nearly enough fiber, vitamins, or minerals from foods, never mind supplements. But because Jenny had not come to me to solve Robert's constipation, I decided to focus on the skin and how his poor diet might be related to the chicken skin.

I asked Jenny more about what Robert drank. "Actually," she said, "Robert is rarely thirsty."

A lack of thirst was my next big clue. These are the clues that I had collected with the help of Jenny's reporting so far:

- dry, patchy skin that presented like bumps under his arms and over his torso

- frequent constipation (though I wasn't yet sure if this was connected to the chicken skin or some other, unrelated problem)

- lack of thirst

What I began to suspect was a deficiency in essential fatty acids. When two very specific fats are not consumed in the diet or through supplements, deficiency symptoms (see page 151 for a complete list of EFA-deficiency symptoms), including chicken skin, will ensue.

KP: BENIGN CHICKEN SKIN OR ESSENTIAL FATTY ACID DEFICIENCY?

If you look up essential fatty acid (EFA) deficiency in a technical nutrition book, there will be a picture of a big patch of chicken skin on someone from a third world country who looks sad and malnourished. The cultural elitism in nutrition education, as evidenced by these kinds of pictures, has consigned malnutrition syndromes to impoverished people in other countries. As a result, EFA deficiency is completely unrecognizable to the average medical professional or misdiagnosed as KP. There is no known medical cause or treatment for KP. What kind of diagnosis has no known cause or treatment? The wrong one. KP is not a diagnosis but a description of a symptom.

The keratosis pilaris support network (www.keratosis-pilaris.org) claims that as many as 50 percent of adults and 50 to 80 percent of adolescents are suffering from mild to severe unsightly chicken skin. One would think that with these numbers, there would be a cure, a telethon, or at least a celebrity spokesperson, but no. Even though the support network says there is no cure for the condition, there is a long list of potentially palliative creams that are supposed to address the symptom without understanding the cause.

Over the years, I have seen minor variations of this presentation dozens of times, and not once had essential fatty acid deficiency been identified as the cause, although the vast majority of cases of chicken skin resolve when the right essential fats are added to the patient's diet.

INTRODUCING THE ESSENTIAL FATS

Most Americans, including Robert, eat plenty of fat, so how can they be deficient in "essential fats"? To fully grasp this very common occurrence, it's necessary to learn a bit more detail about fats themselves.

Fat is a general term for a large group of chemicals that cannot dissolve in water. All fats are made of a string of fatty acids, bonded together in groups. They all have different properties, depending on the fatty acid structure.

Though all cell membranes of the body contain fat, fat is especially important to the brain. Fat makes up 60 percent of our brain, with 25 percent of that fat being docosahexaenoic acid (DHA), the most abundant long-chain fat in the brain and eyes. When the brain does not have enough of this "good" fat, it will develop anyway, but it will rely on lesser-quality fats.

Essential fatty acids (EFAs) are those that the body cannot make on its own; we need to consume them. EFAs are found in nuts, seeds, olive and canola oil, seaweed, and fish. It's always best to eat foods that

---

THE CHEMICAL STRUCTURE OF FATS

(WARNING: CONTAINS TECHNICAL INFORMATION)

Chemically speaking, fats are long chains of carbon molecules. In general, there are two types of fats—saturated and unsaturated. In unsaturated fats, all the carbons are connected by one link (or a single bond). In unsaturated fats, some of the links are double bonds. Imagine a fatty acid as a long section of fencing where most of the posts are connected to each other by either one chain or two chains. The posts are the carbon molecules. Now number the posts in your mind. If the first post with a double chain (double bond) is post number three, that fat is an omega-3 fat. If the first post with a double chain is number six, the fat is an omega-6 fat. But some fence sections are long and some are short. For example, an 18-carbon fat chain (fence section) with more than one double-chain section (polyunsaturated) where the first double bond is carbon number three is called alpha-linolenic acid (ALA). Linoleic acid (LA) is also an 18-carbon chain with more than one double-chain section, but the first double chain starts at carbon

contain the necessary vitamins, minerals, and other essential nutrients, but if that's not happening, then we need to rely on supplements. Essential fatty acids are needed for proper growth in children, particularly for neural development and maturation of sensory systems. Fetuses and breast-fed infants also require an adequate supply of EFAs through the mother's dietary intake.

They are necessary for proper immune function, cognitive development, and function and maintenance of the skin. In fact, lack of availability of EFAs is linked to attention-deficit hyperactivity disorder (ADHD), dyslexia, and a number of other behavioral and psychological disorders. You will find much more about this in the stories about mood and cognition in chapter 16.

There are two EFAs that must be obtained through the diet:

- alpha-linolenic acid (ALA), an omega-3 fat
- linoleic acid (LA), an omega-6 fat

The omega-3 and omega-6 designations have to do with the chemical structure of fats (see the box below). Essential fats are a structural part

number six, so it is an omega-6 fat. If they were 20-carbon fat chains, they would have different names. Because they have more than one unsaturated bond, both fats are called *poly*unsaturated or *many* double-chained (bonded) fats. If there was only one double-chained (bonded) section, the fat would be a monounsaturated fat.

Even though these are the official essential fats, most of your body and your brain can't use them as they are. The brain, for example, being the prima donna it is, prefers them converted to long-chain polyunsaturated fats (LC-PUFA), mainly arachidonic acid (AA) and docosahexaenoic acid (DHA). So you'll hear that 25 percent of the brain is DHA, for example, but if there are not enough essential fats to build sufficient DHA, the brain will not develop optimally. The conversion process, called elongation, requires a number of additional nutrients, such as vitamin B6. The rest of the body uses by-products from essential fats to produce hormonelike substances that regulate all kinds of body functions such as blood pressure, immune response, and inflammation processes. Fatty acid chemistry, although fascinating, is complicated.

of all cell membranes. They are like the bricks in the wall—important to its integrity and function. In this case, the wall we are talking about is the cell wall. Just like a brick wall might function differently from a stucco wall, a cell built with the right balance of essential fat functions differently from a cell built from, say, french-fry fat. French-fry fats are chemically inferior (even if they taste superior!) to the essential fats but they are still in the fat family, so your body will use them in the places it needs fat, if they are all that is available.

One of the jobs of the cell wall is to decide what to let in and what not to let in. The wall should be permeable enough to let in the substances the cell needs but selective enough to keep out toxins or substances that are not essential to that particular cell. Fats from deep-fried foods and other chemically stabilized fats found in many packaged cookies, crackers, and chips changes the permeability of cell walls so they are less stable and selective.

Our bodies and brains take the essential fats and turn them into other important but not essential (because you do not have to eat them directly) fats. These important nonessential fats are called long-chain polyunsaturated fatty acids, or LC-PUFA. The LC-PUFAs most people are familiar with are eicosapentaenoic acid (EPA) and docosahexaenoic acid (DHA). They are the fats found in fish, but your body can make them from essential fats if it has enough of the right vitamins and minerals. Look at Robert's diet and then check out the sources of the essential fats, alpha-linolenic acid and linoleic acid. Notice that none of these—not even peanut butter—was a regular part of Robert's diet. But he did have a lot of processed fat in his diet: chips, crackers, ice cream, and frozen breakfast foods. The problem is that processed fat is not a substitute for essential fat, so even though a diet may be high in total fat, it can be low in essential fats. Remember, you cannot make essential fats, you have to eat them. Think of it as analogous to being thirsty while sitting in a raft surrounded by salt water. Ocean water is not a substitute for essential drinking water, although technically both are water.

NOW MEET THE REST OF THE FAT FAMILIES

You may have noticed that both essential fats are polyunsaturated, but what about the other fats? Fats can be classified by how saturated they are or by the length of their carbon chain (short, medium, or long). Comparing carbon-chain length sounds like a setup for a bad joke, so let's talk about fats in terms of their saturation. Here's a quick breakdown of what you need to know:

There are two main types of fat naturally found in food, plus other types of chemically altered fats added to processed food.

Saturated fat (fats with only single bonds in the carbon chain) are frequently blamed for raising cholesterol levels in your blood. Fats are chains of carbons with single or double chemical bonds. Saturated fats have no double chemical bonds. This type of fat is found mainly in foods that come from animals, such as meats and whole milk and cheeses, but it is also found in palm and coconut oils, and mother's milk. The American Heart Association recommends that saturated fat intake make up less than 10 percent of the total daily intake of calories.

These much maligned fats do have a purpose in the body. Some researchers, including Dr. Mary Enig, an internationally renowned lipid expert, point out that saturated fats constitute 50 percent of cell membranes, enhance the immune system, and lower lipoprotein (a), a substance highly associated with heart disease. The idea that saturated fats are bad and unsaturated are good grossly oversimplifies the role of fats in our health.

Unsaturated fat (fats with at least one double bond in the carbon chain) is the type that, when used to replace saturated fat in the diet, can help lower LDL-cholesterol levels (the "bad" type of cholesterol) without lowering HDL-cholesterol (the "good" type of cholesterol). Unsaturated fats are found in nuts, seeds, and olive and other salad oils (such as safflower).

Hydrogenated and interesterified fats are manufactured, resaturated fatty acids formed when vegetable oils are partially hydrogenated (or restructured) to make the fat more solid. Hydrogenation is a smelly chemical process that after many steps makes the oil more stable so it does not spoil as quickly. Most food producers, under government pressure to remove trans fats, have reduced them or replaced them with new mysterious interesterified fats that also do not seem to spoil, which makes them suspicious. Both fats appear to contribute to type-2 diabetes by increasing blood glucose levels. Trans fats have also been shown to raise LDL ("bad") cholesterol levels. These fats are found in boxed and bagged snacks and processed foods.

How to Read Fish Oil Labels

With all the recent research on the benefits of EFAs and fish oil, there are now many tasty versions on the market. Many, miraculously, do not even taste or smell like fish but like lemon pudding or an orange Creamsicle. These products look the same on the surface, but one will cost twenty dollars and another forty dollars. The difference is often the concentration of the active ingredients (EPA and DHA). For example, if the forty-dollar product has twice the concentration of active ingredient, the cost in terms of active ingredient is the same. The difference is that you will have to take twice as many of the twenty-dollar pills to consume the same amount of active ingredient. In other words, you are paying the same but taking more pills with the cheaper product. Pay attention to the concentration of this typical product.

There are also special features for some products, such as enteric coating to prevent the pill from dissolving in the stomach and reduce fishy burps. These products do not break down until they reach the intestines and are geared toward adults, but let's concentrate on the basic components of the label. They are overwhelming enough.

Here is a real label from a high-quality product that shall remain nameless (on opposite page).

The first piece of important information is the serving size. This label lists the content of one capsule, which fortunately is one serving. But many products have a serving size of two capsules. Many people automatically just take one and think they are getting what is promised on the label.

Calorie count matters to many people, but most fish oil supplements have very few calories. This typical

CORRECTING ROBERT'S EFA DEFICIENCY

The minimum healthy intake for both linolenic (omega-3) and linoleic (omega-6) acid via diet, per adult per day, is 1.5 grams of each. No recommended amount has been established for children.

I suggested that Robert take two teaspoons per day of a concentrated fish oil supplement. I was aiming for at least 1,000 milligrams total of the active ingredients EPA and DHA. The key to reversing a deficiency is using a larger dose, like what is found in the adult version of fish oil supplements and not the kiddie doses found in "gummy" fish oil tablets or products marketed directly to parents for children. A typical gummy fish oil supplement contains about 100 milligrams of DHA. Children's capsule has ten, the amount found in one potato chip. The most critical data is the amount of active ingredients. For fish oil, those are EPA and DHA. This product has a total of 630 milligrams of EPA and DHA, but the amount of total fish oil is 1,200 milligrams. You can see how a consumer might believe they are getting 1,200 milligrams of active ingredient. Every company has a different concentration of active ingredients. In this case, it's about 50 percent concentration. Not every piece of quiche has the same number of ham chunks. If ham chunks are what you are going for, you have to pay attention to the recipe. Look for 50 percent or higher concentration to avoid taking handfuls of pills. The cheaper brands can run at 30 percent, meaning you will get only about 300 milligrams of EPA and DHA in one pill.

Supplement Facts*

Serving Size	1 Softgel
Servings per Container	60

Amount Per Serving

Calories 10   Calories from Fat 10

	% Daily Value
Total Fat 1 g	2%
Saturated Fat 0 g	0%
Polyunsaturated Fat 1 g	*
Monounsaturated Fat 0 g	*
Trans Fat 0 g	*
Fish Oil Concentrate 1200 mg	*
Omega-3 Fatty Acids 630 mg	*
EPA (EICOSAPENTAENOIC ACID) 420 mg	*
DHA (DOCOSAHEXAENOIC ACID) 210 mg	*

*Daily value not established.

OTHER INGREDIENTS: Fish oil concentrate (anchovy and sardine) and mixed natural tocopherols [which is vitamin E being used as a natural preservative]. Contains soybean oil. Softgel consists of gelatin, glycerin, and water.

products may not contain a high enough amount of EFA to reverse an EFA deficiency. The good news is that it is impossible to overdose on essential fatty acids. Your body cannot take in any more than needed, and the rest is not absorbed from the digestive tract and is pooped out in the form of loose stools. If you have questions about adding EFAs to your child's diet, make an appointment with a nutritionist or other health care professional familiar with essential fatty acids.

My basic approach is to correct the deficiency with supplements and then, over time, adjust the diet to include more foods that are natural sources of essential fats. Within two months of taking 1,000 milligrams a day of a combination of EPA and DHA, Robert's stubborn rash was gone for good. Fish oil is a little like digestible WD-40 for the gut, so his bowels got better, too. We increased the essential fats in his diet, but to prevent any recurrence of the rash and to support optimal development, I suggested he continue taking fish oil indefinitely. Fish oils are one of those supplements that are good for almost anyone long term. Jenny was comfortable with this idea and decided to take some herself.

GUESS WHAT REPLACED TRANS FATS?

Keep in mind that EFAs are fragile entities easily destroyed by heat, air, and light. Spoiling fat is a fast way to reduce shelf life (and profits) in baked goods and snacks, so food producers stabilize the fats, using a variety of complex processes so that their cookies can sit on the shelf and still taste fresh six months later. Grandma's homemade cookies, without industrial help, are good for a week, tops. Hydrogenation and other shelf-stabilizing processes change essential fats into completely undesirable entities, like trans fats. Do not depend on premade baked goods or chips as a source of essential fats. A rule of thumb: If it does not spoil, your cells will not like it. Or, if the bacteria won't eat it, you shouldn't, either.

The never-to-be-fully-trusted food industry with great fanfare has removed most trans fats from baked goods and fast foods. The best reconnaissance suggests that interesterified fats have replaced the old trans fats in highly processed baked goods. What are these fats? Chemically altered oils with little

Although Robert didn't seem particularly moody, behavioral issues (including mood swings) can be a symptom of EFA deficiency. (Read more about EFAs and mood in chapter 13.) And his cognitive abilities did not seem to be affected . . . yet. Nobody was noticing attention issues or school problems. Only his skin structure (the "rash") and one neurological function (ability to regulate thirst) were noticeable symptoms. I was glad his mom was on the case early.

EFAs have also been used in many studies to improve learning. In one classic 2005 study called the Oxford Durham Study, children ages five to twelve with coordination problems (estimated to be about 5 percent of students) took fish oil supplements for three months. The kids who took fish oil significantly improved in the areas of reading, spelling, and behavior compared with those who took no fish oil (a placebo). Most parents would happily spoon in omega-3 fats if their child would benefit in just one of those areas.

What about using omega-6 fatty acid supplements to correct a deficiency? These are often derived from evening primrose or borage oils.

---

research attesting to their safety and no long-term health data; they also do not appear on labels. Although the process was developed in the late 1950s, we know little about the effect of consuming significant amounts. I recommend erring on the side of caution and being suspicious of any boxed, frozen, or bagged food with a long shelf life.

At this point, you are likely wondering why there is no testing on interesterified fats and what the heck the Food and Drug Administration is doing if not testing our food. The answer to this question is beyond the scope of this book because it is too upsetting for family audiences. I can only say, in the most calm and loving way, "Get real." Nobody is even monitoring the safety of a common egg let alone keeping up with an industry that is experimenting with new chemicals every day. We expect government agencies to act as watchdogs for an increasingly complex and global food industry on fewer and fewer dollars. It is not going well, as anyone who has turned on a television in the last year can attest. Safeguarding your family's food quality is mostly up to you, the consumer.

BEST ESSENTIAL FATTY ACID FOOD SOURCES

SOURCES OF ALPHA-LINOLENIC ACID (ALA)

- flaxseed oil (1 tablespoon), 7.2 grams
- walnuts (1 oz.), 2.6 grams
- flaxseeds, ground (1 tablespoon), 2.2 grams
- canola oil (1 tablespoon), 1.3 grams
- soybeans (1 cup), .6 grams

THE BEST SOURCES OF OMEGA-6 ESSENTIAL FATS (PER TABLESPOON)

- sunflower oil, 8.9 grams
- corn oil, 7.9 grams
- soybean oil, 6.9 grams
- sesame oil, 5.6 grams
- peanut oil, 4.3 grams
- butter, 3.3 grams
- chicken fat, 2.5 grams
- olive oil*, 1.1 grams

*Contains 10 grams of healthy monounsaturated fats

Borage oil comes from a starflower plant, something you will not likely find at the local nursery or herb section of the grocery store, because it is grown commercially only for the purpose of extracting essential fats. LA is an omega-6 fat and is essential, yet I am mostly talking about adding omega-3 fats, specifically the LC-PUFA ones. In fact, if you are a detail-oriented detective, you will notice that I technically did not use essential fatty acids at all. I used the products the essential fats are turned into, EPA and DHA.

Which fats or combination of fats is "best" are a hotly contested topic in the nutrition world. Suggesting one combination over another opens a huge can of lard, and the nutrition field is littered with the bodies of experts who have fallen on the wrong side of this debate. The wrong side of the debate changes regularly, but clearly the right combination of fats depends on the individual's situation, and there is not one answer for everyone.

Some nutritionists would have used supplemental flaxseed oil, which contains a combination of both essential fats, ALA and LA. Flaxseed oil or another essential fatty acid product made up of a combination of other oils probably would have worked just as well. The choice I made is based on my clinical experience and preference and is not the only answer. I prefer to use the LC-PUFA because, according to a large Tufts University survey, most of us consume ten times as much omega-6 fatty acids as omega-3 fatty acids. That is logical, because omega-6 fats are found in vegetable oils, and most people consume them more than fish and seaweed. The same survey found that 25 percent of the population (which would include Robert) consumes no DHA or EPA omega-3 fats in any given day. Both essential fatty acids and LC-PUFA are important, but because most people consume at least some omega-6 fats and LC-PUFA have useful anti-inflammatory properties that are discussed later, I tend to concentrate on the latter.

> NUTRITION DETECTIVE
> PRINCIPLE #9
>
> **Follow your parental instincts.**
>
> Robert was not suffering from a life-threatening illness, but his condition bugged Jenny, and she thought there was more to it. Rather than sigh in resignation because the diagnoses and prescriptions were not working, she collected more opinions until she found someone who recognized the condition. Don't talk yourself out of getting the help you need because you are being told it is nothing. If you think it is something, keep looking.

CRAFTY WAYS TO INCREASE EFAs IN THE DIET

Whether or not you decide to give your child EFA supplements, improving the diet is always a good idea. The goal: Increase good fats, decrease processed ones.

- Replace your white-flour frozen waffles with those made with whole grains, which have essential fats in the germ. If your child does not like the texture of whole-grain waffles, you can add ground flaxseeds or wheat germ to the batter of homemade waffles. This is a good transition food for children stuck on all-white bread products. Waffle and pancake batter will keep for several days in the refrigerator.

- Offer crunchy seaweed sheets, freeze-dried sugar snap peas, or baked chips for snacks instead of fried corn and potato chips. Baked potato

A GOOD DAY FOR ESSENTIAL FATS

BREAKFAST: Have dinner for breakfast. Start the day with a bowl of rice and beans, have some smoked wild salmon on a bagel, or make some homemade whole-grain pancakes with a heaping tablespoon of ground flaxseeds added to the batter. Add some fruit.

LUNCH: either low-mercury tuna fish (Wild Planet is one brand) or peanut butter/sunflower seed butter on whole-grain bread, along with carrots and pineapple rings.

DINNER: All-American—roasted chicken served with vegetables, and rice drizzled with olive oil.

EXTRA-HEALTHY DINNER: a small portion of low-mercury, sustainably raised fish (see list on page 152), quinoa, braised green beans, and salad with avocado and olive oil dressing.

chips and sugar snap peas are not good sources of EFAs, but by substituting them for the fried snacks, you take out the sources of bad fats. Too many bad fats can actually increase the need for EFA, so this move will improve the fat situation. Seaweed sheets are a great source of EFAs.

- Drizzle pancakes with safflower or sunflower oil instead of butter.

- To avoid eating bad fats in processed foods, keep more fruits and vegetables for snacks instead of boxed crackers and cookies. If you keep washed fruit and cut-up vegetables in the refrigerator, there is a better chance the children will eat them. Teenagers, in particular, will eat food off the floor rather than wash their own fruit. Vegetables can be dipped in salad dressings that contain essential fats to improve their appeal.

- Experiment with different nuts and seeds as snacks. Nuts and seeds are excellent sources of essential fatty acids and can be stored in the freezer to keep them fresh longer. A week in nuts and seeds could be pistachios on Monday, almonds on Tuesday, cashews on Wednesday, pumpkin seeds (available flavored) on Thursday, sunflower seed butter and jelly half sandwich on Friday, walnuts on Saturday, and hummus (made with sesame seed butter) on Sunday.

- Don't forget fish. Canned salmon can turn into salmon salad with a little mayonnaise and cut-up apple pieces and eaten on crackers. Fish sticks are also kid friendly, and some companies now make them without extra processed oils in the coating.

Is Your Child Deficient in Essential Fatty Acids?

The following symptoms of essential fatty acid deficiency may or may not appear together. Robert did not have most of these symptoms, and chicken skin alone is enough to be diagnostic. However, these are other symptoms you should know about. If your child has any of these symptoms, the problem may be essential fatty acid deficiency and may benefit from the addition of essential fats.

☐ Dry, scaly (chicken) skin patches. May look like permanent goose bumps. Often starts behind the arms.

☐ Dry hair with strawlike texture

☐ Excessive earwax buildup or visible earwax

☐ Excessive thirst

☐ Rare or no sense of thirst

☐ Toe walking (Count this if you notice that your child likes to walk on his toes.)

☐ Eating butter or margarine by itself. One child with EFA deficiency would pick up a stick of butter from the table and eat it like a cookie until his mother stopped him.

What to Do

1. For children age three to five, add 500 to 1,000 milligrams of some combination of EPA, DHA, LA, and ALA once a day—make sure it's as much as a gram (1,000 milligrams) of these fatty acids, not just a gram of fish oil. For children five and up consider using at least 1,000 milligrams of combined EPA and DHA. Most infant formulas contain some

added beneficial fats (usually as DHA from seaweed), but if you're considering giving your child under the age of two fatty acid supplements or want to use higher amounts, consult your health care provider first.

Sustainable Omega-3 Fat Food Sources

According to the Center for Science in the Public Interest, these are the best low-mercury/sustainable* food sources of omega-3 fats such as DHA/EPA.

FOOD	TOTAL OMEGA-3s PER COOKED SERVING
salmon (wild-caught from California/Alaska)	2 grams per 4 oz.
trout (farm-raised)	1.2 grams per 3.5 oz
mussels (farm-raised)	.9 grams per 4 oz.
oysters (farm-raised)	.9 grams per 4 oz.
canned sardines	.7 grams per 4 oz.
flounder or sole	.6 grams per 4 oz.
shrimp (wild trap-caught)	.4 grams per 4 oz.
clams (farm-raised)	.3 grams per 4 oz.

*Sustainable is defined as habitat-sparing, nondepleting, and least-wasteful fishing processes.

2. If you give your child more fish oil than he can digest, the side effect will be loose stools or tummy ache. That is the clue that you have gone a little overboard. Do not worry: Some children are more delicate than others, and you have to figure out the dose using trial and error. Wait a few days and try half the original dose.

3. Your grandmother would not recognize today's fish oil. It comes flavored, disguised as pudding, and packaged like gummy candies. Avoid the gummies: They are bad for the teeth and the dosage is low compared with the sugar content. The pudding versions have no fish taste (although some brands have an aftertaste). If you or your child object to the fishy smell of traditional products, consider one of the new pudding-textured versions.

4. Make sure the brand is purified and distilled to remove mercury; this process also gives it a less fishy taste and smell. According to studies, a vast majority of products are distilled and safe.

SEEK UNTIL YOU FIND

If you are unsatisfied with the diagnosis or advice you are given or have lingering questions after visiting your doctor or reading this book, it's always a good idea to get more input and do more research. Rather than accept the status quo, Robert's mother kept digging for information until she was satisfied. It was frustrating and time-consuming, but following her instincts paid off. Many parents inspire me with their tenaciousness and creativity. They find great specialists, useful products, and helpful research because they do not take no for an answer. One mother, whose child refused to take four different fish oil products suggested by various professionals, spent hours on the Internet until she discovered a mild product made in Norway that her child tolerated.

Another mom was concerned about a supplement that I had recommended for her child. She was intrigued by the possibilities and uncovered compelling studies in addition to those I had provided her, which not only convinced her but have been very useful to other families in my practice.

Whatever your situation, follow the detective protocol: Gather the information, ask questions, use your own knowledge, and trust your instincts about your own child.

Kids and Their Many Moods

CHAPTER 10

The Child Who Wouldn't Fall Asleep

A RE YOU OR YOUR CHILD SLEEP DEPRIVED? Have you spent hours a week lying down with your little one, hoping your presence would ease her into slumber land? Or, are you allowing your child to ready herself for sleep by jumping on the bed or wandering around her room for hours every night? For all of you Ferber Method dropouts (and you know who you are), this story is for you.

There is nothing worse than not getting enough sleep. Sleep deprivation has been a favorite form of torture through the centuries because it literally makes people crazy and victims will do almost anything to get some shut-eye. In severe cases, lack of sleep leads to hallucinations and psychosis. For most of the rest of us, too little sleep causes disruption of normal psychological functioning, more frequent illnesses, reduced cognition, and lower productivity. All parents remember "the fog" of the first few months of life with a new baby. But for some, this fogginess can endure well past infancy.

One expects some sleep deprivation with an infant, but what about a child who is six, seven, or eight whose sleep problems affect the entire family? Certainly, kids should not be up until midnight every night. Yet that is exactly what time six-year-old Annabel was falling asleep.

ANNABEL'S SLEEPLESS NIGHTS

Annabel had been adopted from China when she was eighteen months old. Her parents, Peter and Lucy, had married late and thought that parenthood was outside the realm of possibility. Then they learned that China was taking adoption applications from older adults, and much to their delight, they became new parents when they were in their early fifties. They were never happier than when they picked up their shy, tiny daughter at the rural Chinese orphanage. Their friends, who had mostly older or grown children, wondered how Peter and Lucy would handle the trials of caring for a little one at their age. But because Chinese culture encouraged early development of self-care skills and Annabel was already a year and a half old, they had few problems—that is, until bedtime.

Annabel could not settle herself into sleep. No matter how tired she was or what routine her parents set up, she would not fall asleep on her own. She would lie on her bed wide awake until one of her parents lay down with her and coaxed her to sleep.

At first they chalked up her difficulty falling asleep to normal adjustments to a new home. They had remained in contact with the other families who had traveled to China to pick up babies when they did, and most of them reported having some transitional problems, too. As older parents, they were ecstatic over their good fortune and determined to enjoy parenthood in a way younger parents often cannot. Their golden retirement years were going to involve child rearing, so they had better like it! Besides, age had given them perspective, so they were more relaxed than their much younger parenting peers.

THE LIMITS OF FERBERIZING

Dr. Richard Ferber, director of the Center for Pediatric Sleep Disorders at Boston Children's Hospital, outlined specific methods for helping babies soothe themselves to sleep in his bestselling book, *Solve Your Child's Sleep Problems*, originally published in 1985. These techniques are now popularly called *Ferberizing*. Dr. Ferber recommends establishing a routine leading up to sleep, followed by putting the baby down and not picking her up again until morning. When she cries, a parent is supposed to enter the room and verbally comfort her on a prescribed schedule until the baby falls asleep. No picking up or touching is allowed.

Many parents praise the effectiveness of these techniques, and Dr. Ferber is now a cultural icon. But there are many reasons why children do not sleep. And as they get older, the possible causes multiply. Older children can reason enough to worry, for example. Ferberization does not address the mental gyrations that plague people as their minds become more complex. Once the mind is developed cognitively enough to ponder questions about life and death or what to wear to school or whether Mom really loves me, self-soothing becomes more difficult. To go to sleep, the mental noise has to be shut down in deference to the sensory signals of sleepiness. "I will not think about my math test but will relax, clear my mind, and follow the dictates of my internal clock." Right.

Medical problems and biological issues can also be sleep disruptors. Reflux, tummy aches, developmental delays (such as autism), allergies, food reactions, anxiety, and illness can all throw off sleep cycles. Hormone changes (like the ones taking place during puberty and many of the teenage years) also cause problems. The hundreds of millions of dollars spent on sleep medications each year suggests that many people don't easily learn good sleeping skills. Makes you wish "crying it out" worked for everyone.

Everything delighted them, including the coziness of lying down with Annabel as she fell asleep. As she got older, they read Annabel to sleep. So it takes a long time for her to drift off, they told themselves; it is just a toddler phase she will outgrow. She was to be their only child, after all, so they would make the best of it. But her lengthy nighttime ritual and concurrent late sleep time were taking a toll. Nobody was getting enough sleep, and Annabel was increasingly emotional during the day.

159

As Annabel became more verbal, she started talking at different times about being upset and afraid. Lucy would listen patiently, thinking there was a real underlying problem at school or day care to be addressed, but no specific issue could be pinpointed. Over time Lucy concluded that Annabel's moodiness was her exhaustion speaking. Or maybe, someone suggested, Annabel was developing an anxiety disorder. Her parents were so tired themselves that the entire issue was becoming a muddled mess.

The months became years, and Annabel would still cry pitifully if one of them could not spend an hour or more sitting with her until she fell asleep. At that point the novelty had definitely worn off. Often it would take so long for her to calm down that they would fall asleep midsentence while reading to her. They tried everything: snacks before bedtime, no snacks after dinner. They allowed her to wander, and when that did not work, restricted her to her room. They tried strict Ferberizing, spending more time playing with her during the day, simplifying her schedule, moving up her bedtime, and increasing her exercise. Nothing seemed to work. Once, Peter simply lost his temper and yelled that she needed to go to sleep. He felt terrible that night when she cried herself to sleep, but was hopeful the pattern could be broken. They tried more Ferberizing, but instead of learning to self-soothe, Annabel became more agitated and began having tantrums when her parents were not available to help her fall asleep. Sometimes during the day she was so tired, she would fall apart and burst into angry tirades.

FROM BED TO WORSE

As the years slipped by, Annabel blossomed into a bright, engaging child. Her parents adored her and would have enjoyed her even more if she weren't often cranky and irritable. Lucy blamed her sleep issues. Now six, Annabel had to get up early for school, but because of the nightmare bedtime ritual, she would be up until at least ten P.M. and often midnight. Even on the weekends, she woke at 7:00 A.M. on the dot, no

A Short List of Sleep Wreckers

We are a sleep-deprived nation, so many of you may already be familiar with what can disrupt sleep cycles and otherwise interrupt a good night's sleep. Still, you may be surprised by some of the culprits listed below.

- ear infections/ear fluid
- allergies, stuffiness
- headaches
- rashes/itching
- reflux
- gas/bloating
- constipation
- tummy aches
- muscle aches/pain
- overtiredness
- anxiety
- depression
- anger/agitation
- changing the clocks
- medication
- puberty
- hunger
- any illness
- sleep apnea
- low calcium or magnesium intake
- sensory processing disorder
- seizures

matter how late it was when she had finally nodded off. Annabel seemed to be fighting sleep, and her mom and dad were no longer relaxed, older parents but exhausted, ancient-feeling parents.

Lucy and Peter had heard about me from mutual friends and decided to seek my advice. Annabel was still quite small by American standards, and as a long shot, they thought perhaps there was something wrong with her diet. Lucy insisted Annabel's size was "within range" by Chinese standards. I did not have a Chinese growth chart and decided not to push for specifics. She wanted to look at the diet before pursuing the psychological treatments for sleep disorders, and we could start there.

Annabel's diet was fairly good. Her parents cared about food, were conscientious about eating healthfully, and were good cooks. As an only child, Annabel tagged along on visits to museums and Thai restaurants and was served whatever artichoke or hot-and-sour soup dish her parents were consuming. Peter carefully avoided sugar, and Lucy did not have a sweet tooth, so there wasn't much junk food around the house. Annabel's appetite was on the petite side and she did not like meat, but there were no glaring nutrition issues.

Annabel was an academic whiz, according to her parents, and they had no concerns about her cognitive development. Socially she seemed well adjusted; she had many friends, and nobody called her shy (though she had been slow to warm up to people when she first arrived years before). Her medical history was unremarkable except for some sinus infections and seasonal allergies. Allergies can cause stuffiness, making it hard to fall asleep, as any sufferer will concur, so I made a note. Lucy said Annabel took antihistamines as needed.

Annabel had been abandoned as an infant, so there was no prenatal information available. Presumably her time in the womb and first year and a half of life were not nutritionally optimal, so I suggested she take a general multivitamin and some extra zinc. (For more on zinc, see page 116.) Residents of Chinese orphanages tend to eat a diet of porridge and gruel and be small by our standards, so extra nutrition support seemed prudent.

The clues so far were as follows:

- No significant history of medical problems, except seasonal allergies
- No problems with academic or social development. Annabel was at the top of her class and had plenty of friends.
- Unknown prenatal history
- Spent first eighteen months in an institution
- Varied, balanced diet

The only two potential sleep disrupters on this list were allergies and post-institution emotional trauma. I asked Peter and Lucy whether Annabel's sleep issues got better or worse seasonally and they said no, so I ruled out allergies as the cause. The antihistamine Lucy sometimes gave Annabel was known to cause sleepiness as a side effect. No such luck with Annabel.

As for emotional causes, they are trickier to parse. Even if early trauma or anxiety caused Annabel's sleep disturbance, what intervention would change the pattern? This line of inquiry can lead to thousands of dollars of therapy or some scary medicine or both. Deciding the therapy and medicine would be there waiting if other approaches failed, I decided to recommend the path of least intrusion. I suggested a trial of the sleep regulator melatonin.

HELPING THE BRAIN TO SLEEP

Melatonin is a hormone produced by the pineal gland in the brain that is secreted at night to regulate the body's sleep and wake cycles. It is also available as an over-the-counter supplement, and studies have found it to be a safe and effective way to ease children (and adults) into sleep. For children who do not swallow pills, it is available in liquid and melt-tab forms.

Peter and Lucy started giving Annabel .5 milligram of melatonin about an hour before bedtime. It worked the first night. They were stunned. The results are generally rapid, but sometimes the dose has to be increased to 1 milligram. Parents usually know if the dose is correct within a few days, although like everything, there is some trial and error, and some kids may not respond to the melatonin.

Annabel's life changed completely. She became well rested and less cranky. Even at her young

> Melatonin is not habit-forming because it is made in the brain whether you take it or not.

age, she recognized that the melatonin helped her fall asleep, and she reminded her parents if they forgot to give it to her. Melatonin is not habit-forming because it is made in the brain whether you take it or not. Nobody knows why some people sleep better when extra is added. Do they not make enough? Do stress or other factors reduce the amount available or needed? It is some kind of kink in the system with no ready explanation.

In Annabel's case, skipping it meant she went right back to having trouble sleeping. She needed melatonin to fall asleep quickly, but not taking it did not make her worse, because it is not addicting. Her situation was more analogous to needing fiber to go to the bathroom. You normally need fiber to habitually produce BMs. Some people need more fiber than others to have happy bowels, but needing bran for normal BMs does not mean a person is a roughage addict. It's the same with melatonin, except we do not know why some people need more than they make. Many parents in my practice use it as needed or irregularly, and that system works just as well. Every child is different.

MELATONIN: WHAT IT IS AND WHAT IT DOES

Melatonin is a hormone made from the amino acid tryptophan in the pineal gland, a small cone-shaped gland in the middle of the brain. Amino acids are the building blocks of proteins. They are also the building blocks of neurotransmitters, and in this case, a hormone. Tryptophan is converted to the neurotransmitter serotonin, which can be further changed (through the chemical processes of methylation and acetylation, for you scientific types) into the fat-soluble hormone melatonin. The fat-soluble part is significant, because the brain is mostly fat, which means melatonin can float across brain membranes easily.

Release of melatonin follows a circadian rhythm, meaning it rises and falls in a twenty-four-hour pattern controlled by light. At night, pineal activity and melatonin synthesis increases, but once the sun comes up, the levels drop. Nocturnal melatonin levels decrease with puberty and old age, which may account for the rotten sleep patterns of teenagers and their grandparents.

Because studies of neurotypical children taking melatonin have shown promising results with very few side effects, children with neurological issues and developmental delays have been studied, too. Sleep disturbance can be even more problematic in kids with learning difficulties, cerebral palsy, and autism spectrum disorders—perhaps because the neurological issues affecting their developmental delays also affect the part of the brain that reads and sends out sleep signals. I chose to tell

Annabel's story precisely because it is uncomplicated by other medical issues, but I talk about melatonin at least twice a month to parents of children on the autism spectrum or with other developmental delays, and it works just as well for many of them. Melatonin has also been used to treat jet lag and depression and to improve immune function (including reducing cancer risk).

Because melatonin naturally gets turned on at night, taking a small dose as a supplement simply increases the amount available. The sleep signal intensifies, and off you go to dreamland. If it takes more than about twenty minutes to fall asleep, the problem is classified as sleep latency. Taking melatonin is an excellent substitute for counting sheep for those with sleep latency. Unfortunately, waking up in the middle of the night and having trouble falling back to sleep is a whole other can of fairy dust, and melatonin does not work particularly well for that sort of insomnia.

Melatonin has also been found to have promising antiseizure properties. One theory is that melatonin increases the neurotransmitter gamma-aminobutyric acid (GABA). GABA is the primary calming chemical in the brain. The studies have been small, and it is not clear if some seizures may respond better than others. A review of old studies found cases where the hormone may have increased the frequency of epileptic events, raising concerns. If you have questions about melatonin use by children on anticonvulsant medication, bring them up with your child's physician. But ask your doctor before using melatonin in a child with a seizure disorder.

IS THERE A DOWNSIDE?

Annabel's outcome was dramatic, but melatonin is not a panacea for all childhood sleep disorders. There is much we do not understand about sleep. Melatonin works by enhancing a chemical pathway involved in sleep. When a sleep issue is caused by something else, melatonin may not have an effect. The good news is that there are no buildup or toxicity concerns with melatonin. According to the National

Institutes of Health, "based on available studies and clinical use, melatonin is generally regarded as safe in recommended doses for short-term use. Available trials report that overall adverse effects are not significantly more common with melatonin than placebo." This is as close as you are going to get to a government endorsement of safety.

The most common side effect from melatonin is loud dreams or nightmares. In rare cases, melatonin agitates children and seems to keep them up. Some kids are groggy the next morning after taking it, although this can usually be corrected by lowering the dose.

The most common precaution has to do with other medications, specifically those that also act on serotonin (mainly antidepressants). Although selective serotonin reuptake inhibitors (SSRIs) such as fluoxetine (Prozac), Zoloft, and Celexa can be taken with melatonin, they do interact with it, so ask your health care provider about how to use them together safely. Prozac, for example, is thought to lower melatonin levels, so if your child is taking that medication, her need for melatonin may increase. Again, if you have any questions about medication interactions, it's best to consult your child's physician.

IS MELATONIN ADDICTING?

I have not seen a single study directly addressing the question of whether melatonin is addicting, which is unsurprising because there is nothing chemically about melatonin that suggests addiction potential. However, my experience with kids suggests that practically anything can be psychologically addicting to them. If Mr. Blanket or Pooh Bear can be a sleep necessity, why not the ritual of taking melatonin, which in the child's experience has helped her sleep? Adult brains make the same kinds of associations.

If your child still needs regular melatonin help after years of use, ask yourself whether something else is going on. The few times I have been faced with this scenario, I suggested playing the placebo game. This is completely ethical and scientists do it all the time. You can play the game with a small piece of non-name-brand, nonchocolate candy, but I prefer a dissolvable or chewable vitamin B12 tablet (available at any health food store and larger supermarkets with a vitamin section). They look more like a melatonin supplement than a piece of candy. I prefer not to use gummy candies, because I have spent way too many hours at the dentist and do not wish that fate on any child. For youngsters already swallowing pills, you empty their current melatonin capsule and fill it with rice or other flour.

Announce to your young experimental subject that you found a new melatonin flavor you think they will like. Then substitute the placebo. Try not to look guilty. Kids have a spooky ability to spot subterfuge. Usually the placebo works for at least a couple of days and sometimes a couple of weeks, but one night it stops working. The results tend to be obvious. The child mostly does not need the melatonin but sometimes does. Tell the child you agree that the new melatonin does not work as well as the old one, but the fact that he did so well with the inferior melatonin proves he does not need it all the time. "Let's just use it when you are having a tough night. You let me know when you need it." Melatonin appears to be safe enough to use regularly or irregularly for years.

A vast majority of melatonin available in this country is synthetically produced. "Natural" melatonin would have to come from the pineal glands of an animal, and regulations require that plant or animal sources be specified. Check your bottle, but unless it says "contains pig" (just kidding) or lists a source, it is manufactured in the laboratory. Because of concerns about mad cow disease (bovine spongiform encephalopathy) most people prefer nongland sources for this substance.

Consumer Lab, a for-profit organization that monitors supplements (www.consumerlab.com), tested nineteen popular melatonin supplements, and all of them contained the amounts claimed on the bottle and dissolved properly for absorption. There have been few quality-control issues with this particular supplement. Still, talk to your health care professional before giving it to your child. Start with the lowest dose possible (.25 to .5 milligram) and use only as much as you need to get the job done.

NIGHT TERRORS

Some parents come to me when their children wake up in the middle of the night screaming in terror. The parents say they usually jump out of bed, run to their child, and try to wake him. If the child is not awake when screaming, he is probably experiencing what is called night terrors, a sleep problem that affects about 15 percent of kids between the ages of two and six years (though night terrors can occur at almost any age).

In most cases, night terrors are nothing to worry about—although they can scare parents! Typical night terrors last about five to thirty minutes, and afterward children usually return to a regular sleep and don't even remember the episode in the morning. It's best not to try to wake your child during the night terror, but rather gently try to calm him by holding or comforting him.

> **NUTRITION DETECTIVE PRINCIPLE #10**
>
> ## Sometimes you have to think outside the box.
>
> In desperation, Annabel's parents explored the idea that diet might be causing her sleep issues, but I took them in a completely unexpected direction. Melatonin is not a vitamin or a food or a drug. As a result, it does not belong to one specialty and there is no one way to find out about it. You have to run into a doctor, nutritionist, psychotherapist, sleep specialist, or pharmacist who knows how to use it, or you have to think outside the box and try it on your own.

Night terrors are often triggered in children who are overtired, so the best bet for avoiding them is sticking to a good bedtime routine and making sure your child is getting enough rest. If your child gets frequent night terrors, you may want to wake her up before the time she usually has one; this sometimes helps to interrupt or alter the sleep cycle in such a way as to prevent night terrors from occurring. (It also works for sleepwalking.)

- Similar to sleepwalking and sleep-talking, night terrors are thought to happen when a person gets stuck between sleep and arousal. The sufferer is neither deeply asleep nor fully awake.

- Although children usually recall nightmares, they usually don't recall having a night terror.

- Unlike nightmares, night terrors usually occur in the early part of the night, one to four hours after going to sleep.

- Most children outgrow night terrors as they get older.

Does Your Child Have Sleep Issues?

It seems an obvious question that any parent could answer quickly with a yes or no. But many parents grow accustomed to bedtime dysfunction and start to think, "This is just the way it is" or "Lots of kids have trouble falling asleep." Perhaps your child could not be Ferberized and you are too tired to come up with another plan.

☐ Does your child take more than thirty minutes to fall asleep?

☐ Is your child's actual bedtime (i.e., when he falls asleep) later than you would like or later than when you think is best for him?

☐ Does your child get anxious or seemingly more alert as bedtime approaches?

☐ Does your child wake up groggy and tired or have trouble getting up?

☐ Does your child have dips in energy or mood in the middle of the afternoon?

☐ Does your child often come into your bed in the middle of the night, after waking up?

☐ Do you think your child is not getting enough sleep?

☐ Was there a time when your child used to sleep (including going to sleep and sleeping through the night) with ease, but he isn't now?

If you answer yes to three or more of these questions, your child's sleep habits need help.

What to Do

Sleep is complicated, but there are a number of good rules to follow to help your child regulate his sleep—whether or not he's taking melatonin.

1. Set a bedtime; the more regular a child's schedule, the better for his body to reestablish its rhythm and click into its need for sleep.

2. Exercise. Studies don't lie: The more physical activity your child gets during the course of the day, the better he will sleep at night. Timing is important, and exercising right before bed does not work for most children.

3. Stay away from sugar and caffeine; both keep kids awake. This tip may seem like a no-brainer, but sometimes we forget just how sensitive our little gals and guys are to the influence of sugar and anything that might contain caffeine (chocolate ice cream, for instance).

4. Introduce some relaxation exercises:
   - Say good night to your body parts, starting with the toes and moving to the head.
   - Read together. Whether your child enjoys being read to, enjoys reading to you, or finds pleasure reading on his own, this activity calms the brain and distracts children from worries or preoccupations.

5. Consider using melatonin.

Sleep has a huge impact on every function your child is trying to accomplish—from physical growth to management of their emotions to brain development and learning. Thus, it's important to pay attention anytime your child's sleep seems disturbed.

CHAPTER 11

Hyper and Annoying: Otherwise Known as Tyler and Oscar

THE NUMBER OF DISTRACTED AND DISRUPTIVE children in America's classrooms seems to be spiraling up, up, and up. Currently, 4.5 million children (7 percent of the kid population) have a diagnosis of attention-deficit hyperactivity disorder (ADHD). Add learning disabilities and other functioning problems, and the number of children needing special services to get through school climbs to a whopping 18 percent of kids, or one in six.

Gone are the days when Sister Mary Agatha would rap disruptive little Donald on the knuckles with a ruler while the rest of the classroom sat quietly at their desks focusing on the lesson. Now it is more likely that Sister Mary Agatha has several Donalds to cope with in a class of twenty-five to thirty children and is feeling overwhelmed trying to manage. "It will be such a relief to retire," a public school teacher confessed to me while we were chatting at a party. "This year we could not control a boy who kept kicking other children." Three other teachers listening to the conversation jumped in, all sharing similar stories of classrooms overrun with distracted and disruptive students.

"Every year my class seems to be worse," one summed up the situation, and the others nodded in grim agreement.

Donald and his buddies are populating every school in the country, much to the frustration of teachers and other children in the classroom. If you do not have a child at home who could use a speed-control knob so you could turn him down a notch, you certainly know one or your child is coping with one at school. A child like Tyler.

TASMANIAN TYLER

Tyler, age seven, was the eldest of three boys. Cathy, his mother, was a formerly energetic account executive who had morphed into a frazzled self-described "crazy person." Years of dealing with her wild brood, with Tyler being the most trouble, had left her exhausted and stressed out.

Like many hyperactive children, Tyler could be happy and funny, Cathy insisted. He was an idea-a-minute, full-of-life child who could be very charming—but he could also spin out of control in an instant, becoming unbearable. If asked to perform an undesirable task or to stop what he was doing, the Tasmanian devil emerged. He would poke his younger brothers to the point of tears or run around in circles screaming, "Nooooooooooo." His only setting was Warp 9. "He's tiring me out," admitted Cathy, "and he unfairly takes up a disproportionate amount of my time and attention."

Tyler's state of perpetual motion made following directions impossible. When he inevitably made a mistake or did not obey, he would stir up mischief to redirect any scolding. Cathy would be about to have a stern word with Tyler about dumping everything out of the toy closet when her four-year-old would start wailing.

"Mason made a mess," Tyler would say about his brother, affecting an innocent look. Meanwhile the peanut butter sandwich Mason had been happily eating would be inexplicably stuck to the wall.

His school behavior was no better. He talked too loudly and often out of turn. If he could not be first in line or was told no, he would pitch a fit. At least there he had an aide assigned to him to help him keep his hands to himself and redirect him. "I need a full-time shadow myself," Cathy wisecracked.

By the time I met him, Tyler had passed rambunctious and was circling nonfunctioning. Even with a helper, his school thought he was too disruptive and insisted on a full medical evaluation. After a frustrating evaluation session during which Tyler often refused to cooperate, the doctor pronounced him "beyond ADHD," thinking that Tyler's diagnosis might be oppositional defiant disorder or even a mild form of autism because his behavior seemed so debilitating. He recommended Risperdal, a strong medicine for extreme behavioral and mood disorders.

Cathy was expecting a prescription for a stimulant, such as Ritalin. She was unfamiliar with Risperdal, a medication used when children are violent or cannot control their impulses. Cathy knew Tyler was out of control, so she and her husband had to seriously consider putting him on the medication. They also had to weigh the effect of Tyler's behavior on the well-being of their other two children. When she looked up the long list of the drug's side effects, however—which included weight gain, anxiety, fatigue, urinary incontinence, tremors, dizziness, and tardive dyskinesia (uncontrolled movements), she hesitated. She told her husband she wanted to consider some other options first. That's how they found me.

Cathy had heard of me through a colleague of mine, her brother-in-law Jim. I had been hearing stories about Tyler from Jim, too. He had regaled me with horrific anecdotes after visits with his nephews, particularly Tyler. He loved them dearly, but confessed the visits were difficult because the boys were so unruly. "And you should see what they eat," he would say conspiratorially, knowing he had a sympathetic ear. "Would you talk to her?" Jim asked me many times. I assured him several times that I would, but only if Cathy initiated the call. A year passed, Jim moved to another city, and I had not heard from Cathy. Then the doctor weighed in and the phone rang.

Jim had been right about his nephews' diets—they were abysmal. Cathy had avoided tackling her family's nutrition because with everything else she had to do, the task seemed overwhelming. All three of the boys lived on snack foods: sugary cereal or a cereal bar with juice for breakfast; peanut butter crackers, animal crackers, Slush Puppies, dried fruit, ice cream, and yogurt pops were interspersed throughout the rest of the day. One morning, she reported to me, Tyler had a frozen yogurt pop before breakfast.

Because Cathy was so exhausted from trying to manage her sons' bad behavior, she gave in to their requests and did what was easiest in the moment, rather than try to feed them natural, nonprocessed foods that she would have to prepare and they might object to. She was a smart, good mom, and she never intended for her kids' diet to get so out of hand. Although she felt guilty, she did not believe the diet was bad enough to be the cause of Tyler's issues.

Some readers might be feeling a little judgmental after hearing Cathy's story. To an outsider looking in it is so obvious that the problem is the diet, right? Wrong. The doctor who evaluated Tyler never asked a single question about what he consumed. Nobody at his school ever asked about his diet or commented on his lunch. Even the medical community has consistently denied a connection between bad diet and bad behavior, while at the same time insisting a good diet is necessary for proper development. The message seems to be that a good diet is theoretically important for all, but not actually relevant in any particular case.

The obvious big clues occurring together in this situation: rotten diet plus rotten behavior. What remains unknown is whether or not a rotten diet can cause rotten behavior. Just because they happen simultaneously does not mean one begot the other. We all know children who eat poorly and are perfectly well behaved. But Tyler was far from well behaved, so his poor diet became a suspect.

The fact that Tyler's diet consisted of processed boxed and bagged foods with lots of calories but few nutrients meant that he wasn't getting essential nutrients. The amount of added sugar (processed sugar added to food as opposed to sugar occurring naturally, such as in fruit) in his diet was staggering, even by the regular staggering sugar-consumption statistics. The average sugar consumption at this writing is more

High-Fructose Corn Syrup (HFCS)

High-fructose corn syrup is a highly processed chemical derived from corn starch. This corn syrup is not the product from the grocery store used to make pecan pie or dessert for the church picnic. The fructose part is also not like the sugar found in fruit and honey. HFCS is highly concentrated and is metabolized differently from the friendlier products one associates with it. For example, a typical orange contains about 30 percent of its sugar as fructose, whereas HFCS is 80 percent fructose.

The percentage of fructose relative to other sugars in a product changes the way the body deals with the food. All sugars are metabolized differently. Excess intake of any of them can contribute to obesity, but fructose appears to have less effect on curbing appetite compared with other sugars. In other words, you can eat lots more of it before feeling full.

Since HFCS was developed in the 1970s, food manufacturers have gleefully added it to more and more foods because it never spoils and is cheap. Some health advocates note that this is about the same time the American obesity epidemic started and point their fingers at HFCS as a major culprit. The FDA continues to classify HFCS as a benign food additive, but evidence to the contrary is mounting—especially because it is hard to avoid in the average diet.

The most well-known source is soda, but a careful reading of food labels will reveal its presence in everything from commercial cakes to diet salad dressing. Ironically, it is frequently found in low-fat "diet" foods, infant formulas, and kids' juice drinks. Adding a high-calorie additive that does not help the consumer feel full to diet foods, infant formulas, and children's drinks does not sound like a good idea to me. Best to put any product with HFCS in the first five ingredients back on the shelf.

---

than 32 teaspoons of added sugar per person per day, and it has been steadily climbing for decades. High sugar intake has been linked to everything from behavioral issues to obesity and inflammation to possibly heart disease. Inflammation, an immune response to perceived injury, is now believed to be behind most chronic diseases, and sugar plays a huge role in triggering inflammation. Plus, added sugar in food has calories but zero nutrients. Not just a few nutrients, *zero* nutrients above calories. That means every sugar molecule consumed is taking up the space that could be filled with a substance containing protein, fat, vitamins, and minerals—things children need to grow, develop, and function.

Empty calories obviously can cause obesity, but what about children who are not overweight? Nature is not wasteful. Everything you eat is expected to have value, and to get 100 percent function, you need 100 percent of the diet working for you. If 20 percent of your diet is made up of empty sugar calories, then you're operating on 80 percent. By definition, you cannot get 100 percent output (optimal function) from 80 percent input (diet). The Federal Dietary Guidelines recommend choosing low-sugar food and beverages, but they don't specify how much is considered "low." The American Heart Association (www.americanheart. org) has taken the lead in setting guidelines for the prudent upper-limit intake of all added sugars as half of a person's discretionary calorie allowance. There are no guidelines for children except moderation, a murky, misunderstood concept if ever there was one.

Discretionary calorie allowance is defined as the calories left over after all the person's nutrient needs are met from a diet rich in fruits, vegetables, whole grains, low-fat dairy products, lean meats, and fish. Discretionary calories are estimated based on calories needed to maintain weight. Just to let you know how low this number is, for a moderately active woman who needs to consume 1,800 calories a day to maintain her weight, the recommended maximum number of added-sugar calories is 100, assuming the rest of her diet is excellent. That would work out to about one cookie or half of a small candy bar or two-thirds of a can of soda (about a cup) per day. Children, arguably, don't have discretionary calorie allowance. They need every nutrient they can get. However, they would perhaps have a small allowance if the bulk of their diet was whole grains, fruits, vegetables, legumes, and lean protein sources, and if they were active.

I estimated that Tyler was getting only about 40 percent of the nutrients he needed, with most of his calories being empty ones from sugar and other low-nutrient, highly processed foods. And although his diet was much worse than Liam's (whom we met in chapter 7), he was growing. This is a very important observation about individual differences. Here are two different children who are both somewhat malnourished, yet the effects are completely different.

THE CONNECTION BETWEEN SUGAR AND HYPERACTIVITY

Was sugar making Tyler hyperactive? The connection between sugar consumption and hyperactivity has a long, checkered past. Most pediatricians claim there is no connection, and the American Dietary Guidelines echo that sentiment. A closer look at the research suggests a different story. It is true that high sugar intake alone does not appear to cause hyperactivity in most children, BUT—and it is a big *but*—it *is* a factor for some children. There is often a subgroup of children in studies who do respond poorly to sugar. It is just not a majority of children, so the data gets lost in the general findings. Clinically, I certainly see children who get hyperactive from eating too much sugar, and their parents notice also. When you are evaluating one child, it is hard to say whether his hyperactivity is caused by his eating too much sugar or by the fact that he is taking in too few nutrients because his diet contains so many empty calories from sugar. Studies done in juvenile detention centers where the participants could be watched carefully found that improving diets by taking out sweets reduced aggressive and "deviant" behaviors significantly. My bottom line is this: Even if sugar has not been proven to cause aggression and hyperactivity, it certainly cannot hurt to consider improving the diet before adding medication.

Because I understood just how overwhelmed Cathy was, I was reluctant to ask her to make radical changes in her kids' diets right away. Replacing sugar with braised cabbage, whole-grain

SUGAR ALIASES

Just because the ingredients label does not specifically say sugar or high-fructose corn syrup does not mean the product is low in added sweeteners. If two or more of the following items are in the food, sugar may be the most predominant ingredient, even if it is not listed first.

- dextrose
- glucose
- malt syrup
- corn sweetener
- fructose
- maltose
- agave
- fruit juice concentrate
- invert sugar
- sucrose
- honey

177

ARTIFICIAL SWEETENERS (AND YOU THOUGHT SUGAR WAS BAD)

They are commonly called artificial sweeteners, but officially they are noncaloric or nonnutritive sweeteners. Not that sugar is nutritive; we are talking only about calories here. The Food and Drug Administration (FDA) has approved six nonnutritive sweeteners: saccharin, aspartame, sucralose, Acesulfame K, stevia, and neotame. To further confuse consumers, these are marketed under trade names such as Sweet'N Low, Equal, and Truvia. To know which chemical you are ingesting you have to have bionic vision and the ability to read red two-point font on a pink wrapper. None are without controversy, although stevia (Truvia) appears to be the mildest and probably the safest for children. ("Probably" because nobody is going out on a limb and recommending these substances for kids.) Stevia is derived from an herb native to Paraguay, so it is the only one of the lot derived from a natural source. The rest are made in the laboratory.

The most dubious of the lot is aspartame (marketed as NutraSweet, Equal, and SugarTwin). Researcher Robert Walton reviewed 166 studies on aspartame use; 74 of those funded by the aspartame industry itself declared aspartame safe. Ninety-two percent of the remaining independently funded studies identified troubles.

Dr. H. J. Roberts, director of the Palm Beach Institute for Medical Research and an internationally known expert on aspartame, has written extensively about why nobody should use the stuff. He rolled all these troubling side effects into one condition he called "aspartame disease." The symptoms include dizziness, mood changes, vomiting and nausea, memory loss, and fatigue. Symptoms with the strongest proof of a link to aspartame consumption are depression, headaches, cancer, and *increased hunger* (my emphasis).

Increased hunger from a noncaloric sweetener? That cannot be good. Of course, cancer is no picnic, either. Better to leave artificial sweeteners off your child's menu.

---

muffins, and other healthy foods would have been too much. So all I suggested in this first round of treatment was to take all of her kids off all added sugar for two weeks. I told her to think about this as "a mini science experiment" that would last for only fourteen days. (Sometimes it's helpful to think of changes to the diet in time segments; trying something new might not feel as frightening if you know there's an endpoint.)

Because all of her kids' diets were poor, we would deal with the family as a whole.

They could eat fruit, but not fruit juice, dessert items (such as ice cream, cookies, cakes, candy), or packaged food such as cereals and breakfast pastries that contained sugar or a sugar derivative. They could have bread, salad dressings (as if!), or other foods that contained sugar as a minor ingredient. Artificial sweeteners were also nixed. When artificial sweeteners were added to the food supply, manufacturers argued they would reduce consumption of evil sugar. Instead, the opposite happened; sugar consumption went up and continues to do so.

Some studies have suggested that sugar can be addicting just like drugs. There is evidence that sugar consumption can cause the release of opioids (natural painkillers) and dopamine (a neurotransmitter associated with risk taking and excitement). These effects mimic painkillers and stimulants, and scientists have found evidence of craving, bingeing, and withdrawal when animals are given lots of sugar. The fake stuff does not help, because it keeps our taste buds whetted and wanting more sweet flavor.

TYLER TAKES ON THE DIET

Cathy took on the no-sugar diet. Knowing that the food was in the house, she would not be able to stop the kids from eating it, so she threw or gave away all the cookies, boxed cereals, granola bars, and sugary foods. She considered hiding some items but was afraid that in a weak or tired moment she would give in to pressure from Tyler. And she was motivated. If her commitment to the process waned, she reminded herself of the Risperdal side-effect list and got back on track.

She thought the first few days would be traumatic because Tyler ate so few nonsugary foods. Long ago Cathy had given in to his food demands, so when those foods were not in the house, she expected a big explosion that never came. His appetite was always fine and he was willing to go along with the eating trial, although he asked her frequently

---

GETTING MELLOW
WITH MAGNESIUM

Magnesium is a mineral used by the body in more than three hundred processes. These reactions are needed for normal muscle (including the heart) and nerve function as well as immune system operations. Magnesium also helps regulate blood sugar levels and keeps bones strong. The best source of magnesium is green vegetables, such as spinach and chard. Chlorophyll, the substance that makes green vegetables green, is a circular molecule with magnesium in the middle. The next best sources of magnesium are legumes, nuts, seeds, and whole, unrefined grains. White flour products are low in magnesium because the magnesium-rich germ and bran are removed with processing.

When hyperactive children are given magnesium, studies find they often calm down. Magnesium is safe and nontoxic. Once the body has absorbed all it can, the magnesium operates like a laxative (think milk of magnesia) and out it goes. The dose used in one hyperactivity study was 200 milligrams for children aged seven to twelve years. There are quite a few different forms of magnesium, but magnesium oxide, chelate, citrate, and glycinate are all effective.

---

how long the experiment would last. At some level, Tyler knew he was in trouble and was trying the best he could to help himself. I have seen this unexpected cooperation from otherwise uncooperative children too often for it to be anything but some level of understanding on their part.

After two weeks, Tyler was noticeably better and Cathy wanted to continue the diet. Tyler noticed, too, and did not object to enduring, although he wanted to cheat a little. I suggested that she give him a liquid mineral supplement containing 500 milligrams of calcium and 250 milligrams of magnesium because of their calming effect and because Tyler wasn't eating many sources of these nutrients. Dairy products, which he ate rarely, are the main source of calcium in most children's diets, so he wasn't getting much calcium. Magnesium is found in whole grains and vegetables, other foods he did not eat, so his magnesium intake was low, too. Studies have found that blood levels of magnesium are usually low in hyperactive children. Nobody knows exactly why, but perhaps it's because magnesium is found in items that are not overly abundant in most children's diets. Then again, it could be that hyperactive kids somehow are less able to process magnesium or need more of it.

After one month off sugar, Tyler was better still. His brothers, who had been on the same program, were also easier to manage and better behaved. Tyler was still fidgety at school (which was nonetheless an improvement), but at home, Cathy felt encouraged by the positive changes in his behavior. He listened to her, he was calmer and better able to follow directions and control his physical impulses, and he also began to eat better, consuming real food, not just snacks and dessert. Looking at his two brothers, it was clear that Tyler was not the only kid who reacted poorly to sugar. Cathy wanted to keep going for her whole family's sake. "It wasn't a miracle," she said, "but Tyler has also started to sleep better at night."

The teachers at school noticed the improvement, too. Tyler was starting to interact with the other children more appropriately. He had calmed down considerably, and his aide was able to help other students because Tyler did not require her every minute. We decided to go a little further. I suggested that Tyler take fish oil because it has been found in studies to help hyperactivity. I also recommended another supplement geared precisely toward ADHD called DMAE, and asked to see them again in six weeks.

WHAT THE HECK IS DMAE?

DMAE is short for dimethylaminoethanol, a unique nutrient related to choline found in fish, particularly sardines. It is also found in small amounts in human brains. DMAE is thought to protect the integrity of cell membranes and through that process has gained a reputation as an anti-aging agent; it is sometimes included as an ingredient in super-expensive facial creams.

For people with ADHD, DMAE helps cognition and planning by speeding up the production of the neurotransmitter acetylcholine. Neurotransmitters carry messages between nerve cells. There are high

FISH OIL RX

One day your doctor may prescribe fish oil instead of Ritalin for ADHD. Perhaps not this year, but research supporting the use of fish oil for treating hyperactivity, impulsivity, disruptive behavior, and other learning problems is piling up. As quoted in one 2006 study, "Given the safety and general health benefits of fish oil treatment," one investigator wrote, "omega-3 fatty acids offer a promising complementary approach to standard treatments" [for ADHD]. Although not a prescription for fish oil, this is an increasingly common conclusion among researchers and the reason omega-3 fatty acids are being given to children with learning and behavioral issues.

concentrations of acetylcholine in parts of the brain having to do with prioritizing and planning (executive function), movement, and memory.

DMAE was so effective for ADHD in the sixties and seventies that it was dispensed by prescription under the brand name Deanol. In one 1975 study, it worked as well as methylphenidate (Ritalin). The FDA asked for more clinical studies in 1983, and the manufacturer decided that sales would not cover the cost of further studies, so Deanol went off the market, only to reappear over the counter as plain old DMAE.

Now DMAE is an ingredient in many dietary supplements aimed at the ADHD population.

To find a high-quality supplement, look for a company that adheres to Good Manufacturing Practices (GMP). They often brag about this on the label. GMP means the company follows the highest sanitation, process validation, and quality practices promulgated by the FDA. It is a good idea for all supplements that you or your children consume to meet this standard.

The usual dosage of DMAE for children is between 50 and 200 milligrams a day. It has few side effects but may occasionally cause gastrointestinal symptoms or irritability. Stop taking the supplement immediately if these symptoms occur. *DMAE should not be used by people with epilepsy or seizures.* As usual, talk to a qualified health care professional if you have any questions about DMAE.

THE TAMING OF TYLER

A month and a half later, Cathy called to report, "Tyler is doing great! When I call his name, he now says, 'Yeah, Mom? What do you want?'"

He had become regulated enough to be able to control his impulsivity. At school, he was able to sit still and to be more considerate, so his friendships had improved. The teachers and the principal and Cathy got together to figure out whether Tyler still needed his aide. The positive changes were so fast and furious that his teachers were actually worried that they were too good to be true.

Cathy asked me if she could let Tyler and his brothers have a little sugar as a rare treat or for special occasions. As beneficial as a no-sugar diet is, most people find it difficult to sustain over the long haul. Life at home was so much calmer and more pleasant that Cathy did not want to do anything that would bring back the chaos. True, Tyler had been the worst of the group, but he was not the only benefactor of their new dietary lifestyle. We decided to try letting them have small amounts, sparingly, the way sugar is supposed to be consumed. I suggested that she continue not buying juice and other kids' drinks, which are loaded with sugar, but said it was okay every once in a while to give the boys a cookie. But even with the occasional treat, nobody is having anything close to as much sugar as they used to, and Tyler continues to do well without medication.

OREO-LOVING OSCAR

I met Oscar when he was four and a half. He was quite big for his age, but he was still not toilet trained, had separation anxiety, was sensitive to sounds, and was a picky eater. Immature and tending to get in trouble, Oscar also had fear aggression. In other words, when he got scared, he got aggressive. He did not look afraid—he just looked mean. It was also difficult for him to follow social clues—he'd stand too close to kids, talk too loudly. Because he was large for his age, the other kids were extra-afraid of him. He was the classic annoying kid who bothers everyone in class, and his teachers were concerned.

I also learned that there was stress at home. Oscar's father had recently been laid off, so his mother rationalized some of his behavior as a reaction to tension at home. The onset of Oscar's bad behavior started long before his father lost his job, so I was not convinced new emotional stress at home was the culprit. The school was sympathetic to the family's situation, but nonetheless demanded that the parents get help or they would have to "recommend a different placement."

Oscar came to me after completing a psychological evaluation with a developmental psychologist, who then recommended a psychopharmacologist. All these evaluations and appointments were a huge financial burden for a family with an out-of-work provider, and Oscar's mom, Terry, saw the exhausting road leading straight to the same old medications anyway. "This is just an expensive way of forcing me to put my kid on drugs," Terry snapped irritably. She declined to see the psychopharmacologist.

I could not blame her for being frustrated and steered her toward talking about Oscar's diet. Although he'd been a good eater as a baby and a toddler, he'd been sliding downhill since hitting the two-year-old mark, and was now subsisting on sugary cereal and juice in the morning with a laxative for constipation; a bagel, lemonade, fruit, and Oreos for lunch; and gummy bears on frozen yogurt for snacks. For dinner, he might have a yogurt smoothie, cupcake, and juice; chicken fingers and a Popsicle; or a bagel with cream cheese, juice, fruit, and a cookie. He would usually finish the day with another snack of fruit.

This was a lot of foods containing refined sugar and white flour, both of which burn fast and leave most kids irritable and/or hungry soon after eating. Dr. Alan Greene, a pediatrician from California, contends that children are more sensitive to blood sugar fluctuations than adults. As blood sugar falls, there is a compensatory release of adrenaline. Blood sugar can fall quickly in response to eating food that is mostly sugar as protein, fat, and complex carbohydrates burn or are broken down more slowly. Or it can just start dropping slowly after you eat, in anticipation of your next meal. When blood sugar drops to a certain level, which may differ between individuals, you feel hungry. If you get too hungry, the body experiences stress. Adrenaline is a hormone released in response to stress. It is partially responsible for the fight-or-flight response, which makes the heart speed up and the eyes dilate. The theory is that a diet high in refined sugars and flours causes rapid fluctuations in blood sugar, resulting in an adrenaline rush.

An adrenaline rush in a child can look just like some of the behaviors seen in Tyler and Oscar.

We now know there are receptor sites for adrenaline in the amygdala, the part of the brain that regulates mood and aggression. When the amygdala is activated by adrenaline, good judgment tends to fly out the window and

> Some adults and athletes function very well when their adrenaline is flowing, but the same cannot be said about children—they just become hyperactive, impulsive, aggressive, or angry.

aggressive tendencies are exaggerated. Some adults and athletes function very well when their adrenaline is flowing, but the same cannot be said about children. Their brains are not mature enough to modulate their reactions to "fight or flight." They just become hyperactive, impulsive, aggressive, or angry.

So, as we did with Tyler's family, we took Oscar off all added sugar and all juice except what he needed for taking his laxative. He could still have real fruit. A diet high in refined sugar and flour is also short on fiber, so not surprisingly, Oscar was also constipated. As you saw with Sarah, in chapter 8, cranky often travels with constipated, and we would have to eventually work on that if the dietary changes did not take care of it.

Taking away bad foods and adding new foods at the same time is too much for some kids. Some will go on a hunger strike or become hysterical. Given the household trauma of an out-of-work dad, we decided to concentrate on removing the bad foods from Oscar's diet and emphasizing the few good ones he was already eating. We took away the cookies at lunch and gave him cheese sticks. Previously he occasionally would eat a carrot, but now they were a daily snack. Protein was added at breakfast. He liked peanut butter with sunflower seeds, so that was breakfast Monday through Friday, along with sautéed tofu with soy sauce on weekends. We decided on the tofu dish because tofu is high in protein and his mother said Oscar would eat it. Dinner foods for breakfast are always a good idea as far as I am concerned. What preschooler needs energy at 9:00 P.M.? Better to feed them nutrient- and protein-rich foods in the morning.

The new diet contained a lot of peanut butter, carrots, hummus, and apples because they were the only healthy foods in his old diet. We retained them and repeated them often because they were familiar, but I hoped that once he withdrew from the sweets, he might get bored and expand his diet on his own. I also suggested he take a probiotic, fish oil, and a multivitamin to fill in the dietary gaps. (See pages 126 and 182 for more information on choosing a probiotic and fish oil supplements.) Unlike Tyler, Oscar was not signing on to the new program. The carrots sometimes came home in the lunch bag, and some days he refused to eat a meal.

Five weeks later, Oscar was still not eating a wide variety of foods, but he was more organized, less moody, and more balanced. The biggest, most undeniable change was that he started potty-training himself. Apples, carrots, and hummus all contain fiber, and without sugar to fill him up he was eating larger quantities of them. His stools were softer and bulkier, so we assumed he was having an easier time feeling and managing them. Parents often assume children do not "want" to potty train, but in my experience, correcting constipation and diarrhea usually causes a sudden rise in desire. Encouraged, we slowly started introducing new foods such as eggs, chicken, pears, and cucumbers to Oscar's diet. He was resistant to new foods in the first few weeks of the diet, but as time passed, Oscar felt better and tolerated the changes uncharacteristically well.

Terry might have gotten discouraged as the changes took months, but we got some unexpected support from the family dentist. She was extremely enthusiastic about the new no-sugar diet and was extravagant in her praise for Terry and me. Apparently, she was frustrated with her efforts to improve the diets of the pediatric population in her practice. She was so surprised to be face-to-face with a mother willing to take on sugar, long the bane of good oral health, that she put aside her professional persona and went on and on.

"I bow down to the nutritionist! I am over the moon," she reportedly gushed.

A little over the top, I thought when Terry told me the story, but the comments were exactly what was needed to fuel permanent changes. Oscar still had an occasional outburst, but they were few enough not to interfere with making friends. His ready-to-rumble personality slowly dissolved, and because he was less defensive, he was able to interact more appropriately with other children. The school staff was pleased enough with the improvements that they invited him to stay, and the idea of medication was put on hold, permanently, we hoped.

> **NUTRITION DETECTIVE PRINCIPLE #11**
>
> ## When a child is behaving badly, review his diet.
>
> Bad behavior can also be from bad chemistry. This principle applies not only to sugar but to other potential irritants and deficiencies as well. Remember the binary law of nutrition—the problem is usually an irritant or something missing. Sugar creates both situations simultaneously. It can irritate because of its effect on adrenaline and other biochemical processes, and its excessive consumption creates dietary deficiencies.

Is Your Child Eating Too Much Sugar?

The following questions will first help you examine your child's diet to see how much added, processed sugar he or she is really eating. If you think your child is eating too much sugar, she probably is. Write down what your child is eating for several days and take a look.

☐ Does your child drink more than one cup of juice per day?

☐ Does your child drink more than one cup of sweetened milk (such as vanilla or chocolate milk) per day?

☐ Does your child eat sweet treats more than once per day?

☐ Does your child eat sweetened breakfast cereals or toaster pastries?

☐ Does your child pick at the meal but gobble down dessert?

☐ Does your child eat snacks that are mostly cookies and granola bars?

☐ Does your child eat a breakfast that usually involves syrup (such as on French toast or pancakes)?

If you answered yes to one or more of these questions, your instincts are right and your child is eating too much sugar.

Is Your Child Reactive to Sugar?

Now let's figure out if your child is in the subgroup of children who have behavioral reactions to sugar.

☐ Have you ever noticed your child's behavior deteriorate after consuming a lot of sugar, such as after a birthday party or family event?

☐ Does your child beg or throw tantrums for sweets?

☐ Does your child prefer snacking to eating meals? (Snacks are a significant part of a child's nutrition so they need to be real food, not filler—and too often they are sweet.)

☐ Do you have a moody, aggressive, or overly sensitive child who has a poor diet? (If you think your child's diet is poor, trust your instincts.)

Answering yes to any of these questions points to the possibility that your child is a sugar reactor.

What to Do

1. You can radically reduce your child's sugar consumption in one easy step: Stop buying juice and sweet drinks. That's it. A massive government study involving ten thousand people found that one-quarter of their daily calories and half their sugar intake comes from sweet drinks. Instead, offer your child water, flavored unsweetened water, unsweetened tea, or milk (if your child is not reactive).

2. Give your child fruit. There are significantly more nutrients in whole fruit than juice. For example, blueberry juice that has been stored for six months in a bottle has only 25 percent of the special ingredient in fresh or frozen blueberries that helps brain function. The special ingredient is an antioxidant called proanthocyanadin, and it is also the chemical that puts the blue in blueberry.

3. Do a sugar-free diet trial and see if it makes a difference in how your child feels or acts.

   The best way to do a sugar-free diet trial is to take all added sugar and sugar substitutes out of your child's diet for two weeks. Why two weeks? The first week is to get used to the diet and to create a buffer time period in case there are signs of withdrawal. Nobody looks their best when they are withdrawing from something, and studies have found that sugar can be as addicting as heroin. By the end of the second week, you will have had the chance to observe how your child behaves without sugar and will have a baseline for future comparisons. Then, if you still need to be sure whether sugar is an irritant, let your child have a nice big sugar treat and watch what happens.

   Most parents find at least modest differences in behavior. Some parents describe incredible, dramatic differences. As I mentioned, it's hard to sustain a no-added-sugar diet over the long haul. Experiment by occasionally giving your child small amounts of sugar as a treat.

   Can you just cut down on the sugar in your child's diet? Of course you can, but you will not have a no-sugar baseline, and the changes or improvements in your child's health or behavior may not be noticeable enough for you to stay committed to a more healthful diet.

4. Make a commitment to more healthful snacks: bean dips, sandwich halves, different nut butters, salsa and baked chips, apple chips—try anything that is not sweetened and see how it goes. With the exception of white flour products, almost anything that you substitute for sugar will improve the nutrient density of your child's diet.

CHAPTER 12

The Bipolar Child Who Wasn't

"JESSICA IS A MESS," HER MOTHER, Linda, said without preamble. Nine-year-old Jessica had always been a moody child, and her disruptive behavior had plagued her family for years. When she was a preschooler, her parents told themselves that Jessica was immature and would outgrow her temper tantrums and many anxieties. Her teachers at school were not as tolerant. If Jessica did not want to do something, no number of threats or attempts at gentle persuasion would change her mind. One minute she would be happy and cooperative, the next a screeching terror. She could get so angry that she would whack whoever was nearby.

The staff at her nursery school had muddled through by keeping a close eye on her every minute, knowing a benign interaction could go rogue at any time. By the time Jessica reached first grade, her explosive behavior was ruining school for everyone. Her extreme reactions to situations that did not go her way were interfering with social interactions, and as a result, Jessica had no friends. One insightful and tactful therapist observed that Jessica "lacked insight into the effects of her behavior."

JESSICA'S CHAOTIC BEHAVIOR

Before Jessica's parents arrived at my door, many more experts were consulted and all manner of tests run without conclusive result. For the time being, they put Jessica in special education classes to help her with what they thought might be a variant of ADHD with an emphasis on a "disability of self-control." Another professional whom Jessica's mom had consulted labeled Jessica's behavior as oppositional defiant disorder (ODD), and still others suspected bipolar disorder, which was also her father's diagnosis.

A report from the psychologist who had given the family my name mentioned Jessica's disconnect from her emotions and the environment. When she was overwhelmed, she couldn't answer even simple questions. Jessica had few ideas about how to verbally express her emotions but acted out all her bottled-up discomfort by lashing out. "Could physical discomfort be contributing to Jessica's behavior?" the psychologist had questioned in her notes.

A number of the various doctors and specialists had tried to treat Jessica's symptoms with medicines. Unfortunately, Jessica was very sensitive to medication and reacted poorly to many of them. The ADHD medicines all made her moods worse. The selective serotonin reuptake inhibitors (SSRIs), medicines usually used to treat depression or anxiety, had mixed results. Only Prozac, which she had started a year before, appeared to be helping slightly.

By the time Jessica came to see me, the diagnosis had gravitated to bipolar disorder. The medications prescribed by her current psychiatrist had progressed to serious mood-stabilization medications to deal with the hallmark wild temperamental swings associated with the disorder. The latest prescription, Abilify, caused Jessica to gain ten pounds in two months, so it was discontinued. At the time of our appointment she was on a three-drug cocktail, but her mother, Linda, thought only the Prozac was helping by mildly reducing her anxiety.

Why this lengthy preamble to Jessica's case and her arrival at my door? Because this is a tale of how some kids can react quite atypically to

191

foods to which they are intolerant. In Jessica's case, her many behavioral issues, myriad of psychiatric diagnoses leading up to bipolar disorder, and general unease—all by the age of nine—set up quite a mystery.

THE LAST RESORT

A colleague of mine has a line she uses when someone asks her what kind of nutritionist she is. "I am a resort nutritionist," she quips.

Excited at the prospect of meeting a nutritionist from perhaps the Golden Door, Canyon Ranch, or some other fancy spa, they inevitably ask her, "Which resort?" To which she replies dryly, "The last."

I was Jessica and her family's last-resort nutritionist. Linda was burned out. Jessica was the oldest of three children, and her father, Avi, was a handful, too. Despite taking medicine for bipolar disorder, he had anger-management issues and yelled a lot. Linda and Avi had dragged Jessica to every specialist they could think of, including psychiatrists, psychopharmacologists, and developmental specialists. When these failed to successfully treat Jessica's symptoms, they turned to chiropractors and homeopaths. But no one seemed able to help Jessica function any better. Her parents had reached a new low when the special education program that was designed to manage children with emotional and developmental problems wanted Jessica moved somewhere else because her behavior was so volatile and disruptive to the other children. They were running out of drugs to try and places to send her.

As I listened for clues in Jessica's remarkable history, I kept in mind the fact that when mood and behavioral issues are involved, psychiatric diagnostic labels such as "ODD" and "bipolar disorder" are tricky—they often conflict with each other or describe only a small piece of a complex scenario. Besides, *all* of the myriad diagnoses Jessica had been given could not be correct, could they? Because the worst scenarios had been explored, I decided to start with a clean slate of possibilities and not focus on any one psychiatric label.

The first indisputable clue was chronic, long-standing erratic behavior. As clues go, this is a good one. If, and this is a big *if*, nutrition were involved, Jessica either had a serious vitamin deficiency or a common food was causing major irritation. One of the first principles in nutrition science is recognizing the deficiency symptoms of the major critical nutrients. Both thiamin (B1) and niacin (B3) deficiencies, for example, can have emotional disturbance or even dementia as symptoms. However, this level of deficiency is rarely seen in Western countries except in alcoholics. And as bad as adolescent drug and alcohol problems are in this country, I had to assume that this was not the issue for nine-year-old Jessica. So, I started thinking about food reactors.

As is typical, I filled in the rest of her health history and discovered some other significant clues:

- Jessica had had severe reflux the first year of life, and sinus infections and allergy shots until age eight—more hints suggesting that something was irritating her.

- According to her mom, before being put on the Abilify, she was slight and wiry, and often forgot to eat. Now she appeared bloated and puffy.

- I then looked at Jessica's diet: She was the queen of pasta, consuming mostly white food—bagels, sandwiches, and so on. Jessica was rigid about her food preferences just as she was about everything else, and her parents did not want to fight with her about her diet after a long day of other battles. Rigidity in children about food is common, but further questioning revealed an extreme level of inflexibility, bordering on an obsession with pasta and bread.

I homed in on what seemed to be an inconsistency. Although Jessica's diet was full of pasta, bread, and bagels, Linda swore that Jessica often made healthy choices, including fresh fruits and vegetables. This threw me off at first, until I realized Jessica's eating was as erratic as the rest of her behavior. She might ask for something and then pick at it or forget to eat it. Yes, there were some vegetables and fruit in her diet, but the proportions were small compared with the wheat-based bread, pancakes, and pasta.

As we talked further and Linda became more comfortable with me, she mentioned her daughter's intense, constant desire for wheat-based foods. Perhaps she would not eat much or forget after she asked, but she always wanted bread and pasta. Then she would either eat a few bites or the whole serving. To me, the extreme reliance on these foods was a huge

BIPOLAR DISORDER BASICS

Bipolar disorder (BP), also known as manic depression, is a difficult-to-diagnose mood disorder. The word *bipolar* refers to broad swings in mood, from overly happy and energetic to the depths of hopelessness and depression. There are two main types of bipolar disorder, BP1 and BP2, and within them many variants of symptoms, depending on the personality of the afflicted.

Bipolar 1 is recognized by classic big mood swings, from way up to way down. Sometimes the depression and mania happen almost at the same time in a maelstrom of agitation, anxiety, insomnia, loss of focus, and racing thoughts. Bipolar 2 involves affects classified as hypomania or mania light. Some experts claim BP2 can be easily overlooked because it can be misconstrued as general happiness and excitement. How psychiatrists sort all this out is a closely held trade secret, similar to the recipe for Coca-Cola. Jessica acted like someone with bipolar 1 because

of the extreme swings of her moods and destructive nature of her behavior.

BP is no laughing matter for family members trying to live with the sufferer. Nobody wants to be treated during the "up" phase, even though they can be self-destructive. Kids in this phase can live on astonishing little sleep, though their parents cannot. What feels to the sufferer like enthusiasm and excitement can escalate to recklessness, aggression, and a sense of invincibility. As extreme as these criteria sound, seven-year-olds are increasingly receiving diagnoses of bipolar disorder and then prescribed strong medicines to treat it.

I am disheartened when preteens are given diagnoses of bipolar disorder. The usual treatment is complicated drug trials, often accompanied by unacceptable side effects and hospitalizations. If even 25 percent of these children could be stabilized with dietary changes and simple supplements, the reduced suffering and financial savings would be immense.

red flag. It seemed that Jessica's relationship with gluten-based foods seemed addictive in nature, and this was my biggest clue. I had a hunch Jessica's mood disorder was a food disorder.

I recalled certain people I had worked with in the past who literally acted crazy—seemingly consumed by their need to eat pasta and bagels—and wondered if all of Jessica's psychological trouble might be related to her gluten-fueled diet.

HOW CAN YOU TELL IF IT'S CELIAC DISEASE?

I decided to test my theory by sending Jessica back to her doctor for baseline testing to rule out true celiac disease. If the problem was true celiac disease, we would have to be much stricter with the diet than if her problem was gluten sensitivity. The screening tests for celiac disease are not extremely accurate as mentioned earlier, but given the number of professionals monitoring her case, I felt we should follow traditional protocols in case we could find a clear marker. Many kids who are highly reactive to gluten have growth problems and bowel symptoms, including chronic diarrhea. The symptoms of gluten intolerance are the same as celiac disease. You may recall that celiac disease is an autoimmune disease triggered by eating gluten. Classically, the immune system responds to gluten by damaging the intestinal lining. In gluten intolerance, intestinal-lining damage is rarely seen and there are no autoimmune markers.

Bowel complaints had not surfaced when I talked to Linda and Jessica, but I wondered whether she might have a form of celiac disease that showed only neurological symptoms. Researchers are still trying to identify a good screening test for neurological celiac, but it remains elusive. Neurological symptoms have long been associated with celiac disease, but only recently has there been general acceptance that certain forms of celiac disease may be *only* neurological. Typical neurological symptoms include numbness and tingling in the arms, legs, hands, or feet, dizziness, headaches, irritability, difficulty concentrating, depression, anxiety, or more severe symptoms

HARD-TO-BELIEVE-BUT-TRUE SYMPTOMS ASSOCIATED WITH GLUTEN SENSITIVITY

It's hard to believe some of the effects that gluten intolerance can have. If you have even the slightest suspicion that your child may be gluten sensitive, take a look at this almost crazy list to familiarize yourself with the most common symptoms of gluten intolerance in children:

- anemia
- depression
- dermatitis herpetiformis, better known as "itchy rash"
- nonspecific gastrointestinal symptoms
- eczema
- constipation
- gas/bloat
- immune deficiency
- short stature
- delayed puberty
- obesity
- diarrhea
- headaches
- abdominal pain
- joint pain
- dental enamel hypoplasia
- weight loss
- fatigue
- muscle weakness

If your child has one or more of these symptoms and no medical explanation can be found, consider the possibility of gluten intolerance.

The rarer but also possible symptoms of gluten intolerance that it is hoped you will never have to know:

- malignancies
- brain calcifications
- seizures
- schizophrenia
- brain atrophy
- various autoimmune diseases, such as multiple sclerosis
- bone loss (osteoporosis)
- juvenile diabetes
- peripheral neuropathy
- ataxia

such as seizures. This manifestation of celiac disease without bowel symptoms is considered rare, but in my individual practice I have run into numerous cases, so I wonder if *rare* is really accurate. (See page 92 for the more typical signs and symptoms of celiac disease.)

While we waited the several weeks for tests to be ordered and results to come back, I recommended that the whole family go off gluten. With a family of five, there was a high likelihood that at least one more person was going to be gluten intolerant. Besides, Jessica's many issues would prevent the trial from being successful if the suspicious foods were in the house. We could not depend on a spirit of cooperation and self-control, because Jessica did not have either of these abilities. Linda and I both envisioned gigantic temper tantrums while Linda used her body to barricade the refrigerator to prevent gluten infractions. The idea made us both shudder. But Linda and Avi were desperate and willing to go along. Besides, maybe the diet would help Avi, too.

When it comes to food intolerance, I am a big believer in the old saying "The apple does not fall far from the tree." If gluten was disrupting Jessica to the point of mental illness, one of her parents had likely passed on a susceptible gene. Not everyone is this reactive to gluten, and the tendency is genetic. Whenever I mention this possibility to a family, the prime suspect is immediately identified. The parents will hem and haw about a child, but if I ask which one of them might also be gluten sensitive, the suspected carrier steps forward, and this was again the case with Avi and Linda. Jessica's behaviors were more severe versions of Avi's anger control issues. He, too, agreed to go along with the no-gluten diet.

> When it comes to food intolerance, I am a big believer in the old saying "The apple does not fall far from the tree."

Because Jessica did not have stomach symptoms, I did not suggest removing lactose-containing foods as I did for Shane, in chapter 6. But I did recommend a modest supplement program to close the gaps in Jessica's diet: I suggested she take fish oil (to help rebuild the nervous system and balance her mood; for more on this, see page 182), probiotics (to rebuild her gut; for more about this, see page 126), and a multivitamin (to round out her nutritional needs).

Just as I was plotting a strategy for persuading the family to continue the trial no matter what the gluten screening tests found, Linda suddenly remembered to tell me about Jessica's frequent stomach complaints and occasional bowel accidents. You would have thought that these notable symptoms would have come up during our first conversation (especially since I had asked specifically about stomach symptoms), but they hadn't.

This phenomenon of omitting important information is exceedingly common in complex cases. Bowel accidents and other such incidents often become a forgettable inconvenience compared with the trauma of everyday behavior. Or, if the person happened to not have a particular symptom during the week before we meet, they "forget" to mention that they ever had it.

THE WACKY WORLD OF GLUTEN-SENSITIVITY SCREENING TESTS

If you or your doctor suspects that your child has full-blown celiac disease, consult a gastrointestinal specialist. She will usually start with a group of blood screening tests. The tests have complicated names but basically are looking for ways your immune system is reacting poorly to the presence of gluten proteins. To understand the tests, you need to know a little about how the immune system works.

The immune system has many different kinds of cells and proteins so it can protect your body from all kinds of attacks. The proteins that can potentially react to gluten are called immunoglobulins (Ig). There are five groups of immunoglobulins that are named after the letters *G, A, M, E, D*. Their full names are immunoglobulin G (IgG), immunoglobulin A (IgA), and so on. Each group or family has a different function. For example, IgA mainly operates in secretions or in epithelial tissue lining the gut and lungs. Think of the groups like the army, navy, air force, and marines. They are all branches of the military protecting certain areas of your body in specific ways. IgG is like the army and IgA is like the navy. You need to know only about IgG and IgA for this discussion on gluten.

Immunoglobulins do not always react to gluten, because some people's bodies do not see gluten as an enemy. Other people's immune systems will identify gluten as a problem and start building up immunoglobulins A (the navy) and G (the army). Why some people do this and others don't probably has to do with a combination of genetic and environmental factors.

Immunoglobulins are sometimes also referred to as antibodies. They operate by binding to a suspected problem molecule (called an antigen). The antigen in this case will be gluten. The presence of an antigen is supposed to increase the levels of antibodies. You can tell if you are reacting to gluten because the anti-gliadin (gluten) antibodies from either IgA and IgG go up. Therefore, the screening tests for celiac always look for the following:

- IgA anti-gliadin antibodies   *Translation:* the navy fighting gluten
- IgG anti-gliadin antibodies   *Translation:* the army fighting gluten

The other screening tests also look at different antibodies against gluten. In addition to the two above, the tests include:

- IgA anti-endomysial antibodies (EMA)
- Anti-tissue transglutaminase (tTG) antibodies
- Total IgA levels

Now here comes the tricky part. Notice that we are measuring the total IgA levels. In other words, we want to see how many total troops are in our navy. This is important, because if the total number of troops is too low, there will not be enough to respond to a gluten assault and the other test results will not be accurate. I call this the Hurricane Katrina problem. After Hurricane Katrina, there was a crisis, but there were not enough military personnel to respond. These blood tests are measuring the immune response to a potential gluten crisis, so there have to be enough troops to be counted. In addition to having enough IgA for the screening tests to be accurate, the patient must be eating gluten before the blood is drawn.

Your doctor may add other measurements, such as a celiac genetic test, to the above screening tests. Some specialists also check for anemia, because gluten intolerance causes malabsorption of nutrients, such as iron. Low iron availability can lead to anemia. Flunk a few of these tests and you will progress to endoscopy, the test in which the tube goes down the throat to the small intestine, where little snips of tissue are collected. In celiac disease, the little fingerlike projections lining the gastrointestinal tract, called villa, flatten out. The biopsy sample is looking for missing or flattened villa. Endoscopy with biopsy is the gold standard for diagnosing celiac disease, but does not work for gluten sensitivity because the villa are not affected. A physical marker in the gut for gluten sensitivity has not yet been found.

When Jessica's celiac screening tests came back, her physician interpreted them as negative, although there was a mildly elevated marker for one of the parameters. That marker was IgG anti-gliadin antibodies. Still, that was not enough to diagnose celiac disease. Until better evaluating techniques are developed, the best test for gluten reactions that are not celiac disease is a dietary elimination trial. Luckily, Jessica's family was committed to trying the diet.

THE REAL JESSICA EMERGES

Jessica was initially resistant to this new diet, but surprisingly, agreed to a month-long trial. She was coherent enough to know she was in desperate shape and didn't want to be moved to yet another school. Her mother bought all sorts of gluten-free versions of familiar food. She stocked up on gluten-free pastas, breads, waffles, and cookies, hoping Jessica and the rest of the family would like some of them. Being an organized sort, Linda made a master list of the acceptable and tasty products as they discovered them so she would not forget.

Jessica hung in through a short period of withdrawal from the gluten, which, like withdrawal from anything, can be uncomfortable—physically and emotionally. She was cranky and waspish for several days, but her level of emotional distress was so high already that nobody but her mother noticed a difference. Food-withdrawal symptoms vary greatly from person to person. Some children have no uncomfortable transition. Others fuss or cry easily from a few days up to a few weeks. Long withdrawal periods are rare in children, and Jessica experienced only a few days of intense cravings and emotional distress. The rest of the family had no complaints, because while the house was gluten-free, Linda was not focusing on what the other children ate at school, outings, or friends' homes. Her hands were full monitoring Jessica and making sure there was tasty gluten-free food available for every occasion. Avi, being an adult, stayed strictly on the diet with Jessica and had no problems.

Two months later, Jessica's mother called me and said, "It's amazing. Jessica is a different child. She's calm, smiling, and all the weird behaviors are gone. But all of us seem to be impacted. My husband is more stable with his moods, and my other daughter's eczema went away."

The improvement after one month had been so startling that they had continued into a second

> ## NUTRITION DETECTIVE PRINCIPLE #12
>
> ## Treat the person, not the test.
>
> Tests are great detective tools, but you cannot always depend on them to solve the case. For Jessica, testing showed only mild reactions to gluten, but if her parents had not looked beyond that finding, Jessica would have continued to be treated for mental illness. The best way to find out whether a suspected irritant is actually bothering someone is by eliminating it from the diet. Either the irritating symptoms go away or they do not, and you have your answer. Good medical investigators use tests to clarify the clinical picture. But as a parent, you cannot always rely on tests, especially if what's in front of you does not match the test results.

month. By the end of month two, Jessica's psychiatrist was on board and already reducing her medication. "This is mind-blowing," Linda reported.

In four months, Jessica had reduced her medicines to a small dose of Prozac and seasonal allergy pills. She had woken up like Rip Van Winkle to a whole new world. She literally had years of catching up to do. Sometimes she just did not know what to do with her new self. As a result, she remained anxious, although for completely different reasons than before.

There were many bumps along the road to recovery. Because Jessica's relationship to gluten was addictlike in its intensity, it took her about six months to permanently change her behavior. In fact, sometime during the second gluten-free month she started to obsess about the idea of eating a bagel. Linda decided to let her have one so they could both see what would happen. Almost immediately, Jessica's behavior became erratic and her wild mood swings returned and retraumatized the entire family, including Jessica. Thankfully, she recognized that her behavior and thinking were out of control, and from that day forward she refused to eat any gluten. For a child who reportedly had little self-awareness or the ability to connect her actions to consequences, this was most significant. Jessica had the presence of mind to connect the dots because of this experience: She wanted control over her emotions, and she was committed to staying gluten-free.

Jessica did not have celiac disease but was clearly very reactive, so the question became, How strict should she be with the diet? Should every salad dressing label be perused for gluten derivatives? The answer to these questions varies from individual to individual, depending on how much of an effect tiny amounts of gluten have. Linda decided a cleaner diet worked best for Jessica; she read every label and removed all traces of gluten.

This family was so transformed by this experience that Linda changed her career and became a health coach so she could motivate others to make the kind of life-changing shifts she had experienced. By age eleven, Jessica was an A student in regular classes. Soon after, I was giving a talk in Boston, where Jessica and her family lived. A jovial, burly man came up to me afterward and gave me a big hug. "You changed my life," he boomed. When he saw the look of confusion in my face, he introduced himself as Jessica's father. "My kids think they have a new father," he said. "I am no longer angry all the time."

Is Your Child Gluten Intolerant?

The symptoms of gluten intolerance can vary widely, as I've mentioned several times. So if you are suspicious, trust your instincts—you are probably on to something. To review the possible symptoms of gluten sensitivity, answer these questions:

☐ Does your child have eczema or a persistent itchy rash?

☐ Does your child have "generalized digestive symptoms" such as diarrhea, gas, bloat, abdominal pain, or constipation that have resisted treatment?

☐ Does your child wake up moody on some days and seemingly fine on other days, leaving you constantly wondering what kind of day you will have?

☐ Does your child show a strong attachment to gluten-based foods? Does he have cravings for bread or pasta?

☐ Does your child have extreme behavior problems that are baffling your medical professionals?

☐ Does your child suffer from frequent headaches or joint pain?

☐ Is your child chronically anemic?

☐ Does your child have trouble with not gaining weight despite eating enough?

☐ Does your child have an insatiable appetite?

☐ Does your child have bone loss?

If you answered yes to one or more of these questions, continue reading.

What to Do

1. Familiarize yourself with the range of possible symptoms of gluten intolerance.

2. Consider doing the celiac screening tests mentioned earlier in this chapter. If any of the test results are positive, there is likely gluten sensitivity and possibly celiac disease.

3. Even if the test is negative, try a six-week gluten-free diet. If your child's symptoms (any of the above) begin to abate or disappear completely, then you've discovered that despite a negative test, your child is reactive to gluten and should avoid it.

4. If full-blown celiac disease is suspected, consult a gastrointestinal specialist for further testing and advice.

5. If your child tests positive for celiac, then the only treatment is a strict, gluten-free diet.

JESSICA, THE TEENAGE YEARS

A few years passed, and Jessica asked her mom if she could talk with me because she had questions about her gluten-free diet. Jessica wanted to understand how strict she had to be on her diet and what her long-term prognosis was so she could be more independent while controlling her diet. At twelve years old, Jessica was poised and talkative. She was doing well in a regular school despite some lingering attention issues. Not a single concern on the detailed memo from the psychologist was relevant anymore. The report had claimed that she was a child who could not easily communicate what she was thinking or feeling unless it was in extremes, and cited examples of pathological emotional immaturity. Looking at the young woman in front of me, the memo seemed almost surreal.

Three more years passed, and when Jessica was fifteen, Linda called me again. Jessica was an active teenager with friends. She had allergy and sinus issues to discuss this round, but Linda also wanted to talk about anxiety. Linda was wondering if maybe we could do more with nutrition to address some of the anxieties of adolescence. Linda and I marveled at how far Jessica had come. What a relief to be talking about plain old teenage angst! There are no dietary changes that will cure that, but to learn more about nutrition and anxiety, read on.

CHAPTER 13

The Worrier

U NTIL THIS POINT, THE CASES I've presented have required pretty straightforward nutrition detective work. The emphasis has been on:

- finding clues by hearing a child's history, learning his eating habits, tracking his responses to other treatments;
- piecing data together to form a picture of what's going on;
- figuring out what the underlying problem is and taking steps to remedy it.

In this chapter, the child's problem does not have an obvious dietary link, which makes this, in my opinion, even more interesting, advanced detective work. You will notice that I have tried to creatively synthesize emerging research, my own knowledge, and a burning desire to fill in the blanks to craft an innovative plan that could help alleviate or solve the problem while we wait for science to come up with the "real" answer. Of course, *that* could take forever, and we don't have forever when it comes to our kids' health and well-being.

When presented with a complex predicament with no specific

research pointing to a clear-cut solution, my first thought is, "I wonder if I can borrow what we know about something similar to solve this problem." For example, because the scientific research on children and nutritional treatments is thin compared with what is established about the elderly, I often ask myself if a substance that works well at the end of life when people are more delicate might work as well at the beginning. The next three stories are about out-of-the-box nutritional approaches to complicated problems with unknown or unsatisfactory treatment protocols.

EVIE, THE WORRIER

Eleven-year-old Evie was a worrier. She worried about what to wear to school and whether she did what the teacher wanted on her homework assignment. Her friendships generated endless causes for concern, even more than for your average adolescent girl. She ruminated over everything, from schedule changes to dying. Her brain hopped from one worry to the next, with short breaks of blessed contentment few and far between.

SSRIs and Children

There are about a half dozen SSRI drugs on the market today, but only two—fluoxetine (Prozac) and escitalopram (Lexapro)—are approved for the treatment of depression and other psychiatric disorders in children. Nonetheless, doctors continue to use more than the two approved drugs with children. The National Institute of Mental Health estimates that about 5 percent of adolescents have a major depressive disorder. Many of these increasingly medicated teenagers suffer from one of the numerous SSRI side effects. The list includes dry mouth, nausea, restlessness, insomnia, nervousness, headache, diarrhea, and agitation. For an already depressed adolescent, these are troublesome, but by far the biggest point of contention is the rising number of suicides in the medicated-kid population. People with depression are more likely to kill themselves, but teenagers arguably are more impulsive and try more often. Put the combination of depression and teenage brain together, and a disturbing question arises: Was the mental illness responsible for the suicide or was increased use of medication making vulnerable kids suicidal?

Controversy has ensued. Not surprisingly, the drug industry

According to Cheryl, her mom, Evie had always been sensitive—she was one of those babies who had startled easily, cried if there was a change in the predictable schedule, and reacted intensely to transitions in general. For Cheryl, Evie always needed a lot of hand-holding and help through her days, and even so, often melted down or collapsed in exhaustion by evening. Cheryl was worn out from constantly trying to help Evie manage her low tolerance for the bumps of life and what had in recent years become full-blown anxiety. Although her meltdowns had become less frequent as she got older (Evie was able to hold herself together at school), she often ended the day in a heap of frustration and exhaustion.

In fact, Evie's anxiety had been so stressful for her entire extended family that her parents and pediatrician decided that she would benefit from taking Prozac, a selective serotonin reuptake inhibitor (SSRI), which is the most popular class of drugs used to treat depression and anxiety. The medicine helped noticeably, but Evie still struggled to the degree that Cheryl felt she needed to continue to look for answers.

came down firmly on the side of the benefits of antidepressant medication outweighing the risks. Other consumer and professional groups advise caution. The Center for Science in the Public Interest, a consumer advocacy group that reviews the scientific literature on health- and nutrition-related issues, published a position paper on the subject. A review of fifteen placebo-controlled clinical trials looking at SSRI use in children discovered that only three established that the drugs worked. The Food and Drug Administration approval for the use of fluoxetine (Prozac) in children was based on the positive findings of only two (of these three) studies. The third positive study was for a different SSRI drug. The remaining twelve clinical trials rated the drugs equivalent to a placebo. In other words, they worked the same as taking a sugar pill.

The result of these initial studies is a bunch of mushy, carefully worded warnings about weighing the severity of the illness against the risks of the medication with the help and careful monitoring of a qualified physician. You almost want to add "Blah, blah, blah." Not very reassuring to parents who have been told their child suffers from anxiety or excess worry.

GROWING UP NERVOUS

When I met Evie and Cheryl, they were both nervous. I understood their predicament: a well-meaning parent who was doing her best to help a needy kid by dragging her to yet another professional. Evie was a people pleaser and was trying to manage her fear of meeting a new person. Cheryl was worried I would think something was wrong with her for complaining about a kid who, during the interview, would appear practically perfect. Evie would be polite, calm, and agreeable, Cheryl assured me. She was aware that professionals who work with kids tend to see anxious children as the product of neurotic parents. While visiting the therapist or at school, the allegedly fretful offspring can be easy and delightful, but at home the smallest trigger—such as not being able to find the pants she planned to wear—could start an international incident. Evie knew that she saved the craziness for Mom, and Cheryl was not sure I would believe how bad their home life was; thus two nervous people sat before me.

A few minutes into the conversation, they both started to relax. Evie recognized her anxiety and didn't like how she flip-flopped so quickly from calm to frenzied. Years of psychotherapy had sharpened her awareness, and she tried to use the tools she had accumulated to rationally work through her emotions, but all too often she felt she was battling an unruly brain and the brain was winning. "Everything is such a big deal," she confessed. A smart kid who wanted to know more, Evie was motivated to "feel normal."

Cheryl nodded in silent agreement, although she was reluctant to comment with Evie present. Instead, she had sent me a long note in advance of our meeting, which allowed me to fill in the details of the story from the pieces Evie was willing to disclose. In that note, Cheryl had confided that she was perimenopausal, and she felt that was contributing to her thinning patience. It's also significant to note that Evie, at age eleven, was closing in on puberty, which with its hormonal swings could make the situation only more difficult. Hormonal changes make people more sensitive because hormones communicate with neurotransmitters and affect

LIVING WITH AN ANXIOUS SIBLING

Extreme anxiety is not just hard on the sufferer and her parents. It's hard on siblings and friends, too. Skylar, a teenager who is not a worrier, grew up with an older sister, Nadia, who was plagued with generalized anxiety. "When I was little, I didn't really notice," Skylar explains, "but as I got older, I understood." Interactions with her older sister were something to dread. "She constantly asks for my advice, and the discussion is always about her, because she is always stressed out about stuff," she continues. "But then she asks everyone, gets different advice, and is more stressed out than ever."

The strain on the family comes from the inability of anyone to calm Nadia down, despite massive efforts. "She just swings," Skylar says flatly. According to Skylar, Nadia is needy one minute and screaming, "You don't help me with anything" the next.

"You have to know your boundaries," Skylar intones sagely, belying her tender years. "I have gotten really good at talking to people." Playing to her hard-learned strengths, Skylar thinks she may one day pursue a career in counseling or arbitration. "I always sound just like this no matter how upset people are," she says with surreal calm, and I wonder if that is a good thing.

---

brain operations. Evie and her mom were turning up in my office now because they were hitting the hormonal tipping point. Cheryl had heard through word of mouth that I used nutrition creatively to help the brain, and she was hoping there was a magic vitamin that might help her daughter.

After hearing about Evie's situation, I asked her about what she ate. Although I could have gathered this information from her mom, I thought that at age eleven, it would be helpful for Evie to become more aware of what she was eating. I learned that she was actually a pretty good eater. She ate a lot of fruits and vegetables, chicken, yogurt, and even some whole grains, such as seven-grain bread. She had occasional treats, but not a lot of junk food.

Then I turned to Cheryl and wanted to know more about Evie's health in her early life. I asked a lot of questions about her immune system. Was she sick a lot? Did she have frequent ear infections? How was her digestion and elimination? Did she seem allergic to anything? Did she eat well as a baby and toddler?

I learned that there was nothing notable beyond fussiness and sensitivity to loud noises, which started at birth. Otherwise, she had a normal number of mild childhood illnesses but no pattern of problems and no other ongoing medical issues. I was not questioning the accuracy of the anxiety diagnosis, but wanted to see if there were other clues with nutritional links. According to wrongdiagnosis.com, almost any symptom, such as anxiety, could have from a handful to thousands of possible causes. This fascinating site (which should be avoided by hypochondriacs) tells you hundreds of other conditions you might have, depending on your spectrum of symptoms. The more symptoms you input, the further the potential list of diagnoses gets whittled down. Practitioners in different fields run down similar lists in their heads as the starting point for considering other possibilities.

I went through a mini-version of wrongdiagnosis.com in my own mind using my experience and training, and asked myself what could be the possible causes of Evie's symptom of anxiety:

- a food sensitivity?
- a sleep disturbance?
- a nutrient deficiency?
- sensory processing disorder?

These were the most common reasons for anxiety that came to mind. If Evie had one of these, I could determine the direction nutrition therapy should take. But alas, a well-traveled path was not to be. Evie did not have symptoms of food intolerances (such as digestive complaints or a rash) and slept like a baby. Her diet was excellent, and there was no glaring nutrient deficiency to pursue.

Sensory processing disorder (SPD) occurs when the nervous system does not mature evenly and in a timely manner. The result is difficulty taking in or interpreting information received through sight, sound, touch, tastes, smells, and movement. People with SPD are often anxious because what they perceive overwhelms them, and life feels out of control. For example, sounds are too loud, lights are too bright, and touch is too invasive. Getting through the day feels like navigating a minefield of painful sensations, and the sufferer is worried about what will assault them next. See chapter 17 for more about nutrition and SPD. But Evie did not have enough symptoms on the SPD checklist to make that diagnosis.

With no obvious cause to direct a course of action, I started thinking about the nutritional supplements geared toward anxiety.

AMINO ACIDS AND ANXIETY

There are many nutritional supplements geared toward anxiety. The most popular has a specific amino acid (the basic building material of proteins) as the active ingredient. Neurotransmitters are the chemicals that allow one nerve cell (neuron) to talk to muscle, a gland cell, or another nerve. They are released or transmitted from the end of a nerve cell and the message is delivered to the target cell. Most neurotransmitters are made from amino acids. Tyrosine can become the neurotransmitter dopamine, and tryptophan can be used to build serotonin, for example. In theory, loading up on the amino acid needed to make the neurotransmitter you need more of should help favorably increase neurotransmission in that part of the brain. Some antianxiety supplements contain an amino acid, like tryptophan, plus vitamins and minerals needed to turn the amino acid into the desired neurotransmitter. In rare cases, notably gamma-aminobutyric acid (GABA), which is the primary calming chemical in the brain, the product is the neurotransmitter.

How do neurotransmitters work? There are microscopic spaces (synapses) separating cells, and neurotransmitters are the chemicals that communicate in these spaces. Although we think of neurotransmitters as being only in the brain or communicating between nerve cells, they actually operate all over the body when one cell wants to communicate with another. Scientists do not understand the precise mechanism of each neurotransmitter or even how many exist.

What we do know is that if cell A wants to send a message to cell B, it has to release a neurotransmitter, which crosses the synapse and docks into a receptor site in cell B. The receptor determines the message by accepting the communication; the neurotransmitter's only job is to activate one or more receptor. It is like texting but faster.

There are different types of receptors. Some send messages that excite the neurons, and some send messages that inhibit or slow down the neurons. Each neurotransmitter has a specific affinity for a type of receptor, but some neurotransmitters connect with a variety of receptors. For example, acetylcholine, a neurotransmitter important for motor functions, binds to both excitatory and inhibitory receptors. When one takes into consideration more than a hundred different neurotransmitters, all with varying affinities to a number of types of receptors, and factors in different concentrations of each neurotransmitter controlling a multitude of processes, the result is a very complicated system.

Within this interconnected galaxy, nutritional products designed to support neurotransmitters can be extremely effective or worthless, depending on many known and unknown factors. If you want to enhance serotonin, for example, you can take 5 hydroxytryptophan (5HTP), a form of the amino acid tryptophan that is directly converted to serotonin. That should increase the available serotonin, right? But wait, other nutrients are also needed to effect that process, and in addition, the rest of the diet has to support absorption of the tryptophan. Furthermore, you have to consider the processing of the serotonin in the synapse, which nutrients may not affect, and serotonin's ability to bind to the target neuron, which seems to also be affected by exercise. If you're still with me, you're likely thinking, MAYDAY, BRAIN OVERLOAD! As you can see, brain chemistry is way more complicated than simply popping a supplement. (And those are just the factors we know about.)

When you hit the right pathway just so, the angels sing and life improves. Miss and nothing happens, or undesired side effects ensue because the neurotransmitters in the brain talk to each other, and you might have inadvertently sent the wrong message. Unfortunately, we do not fully understand the chemical language of anxiety—far from it. We do not know if the biochemistry of generalized anxiety disorder is the same as post-traumatic stress disorder, for example. According to the Child Anxiety Network, there are many types of childhood anxiety: generalized anxiety disorder, panic disorder, separation anxiety disorder, specific phobias, selective mutism (a condition where a person is able to speak most of the time, but not in certain situations), social phobia, obsessive-compulsive disorder, and post-traumatic stress disorder. Despite this wide variety of causes and the myriad nuances between conditions, medically they are all treated with some combination of SSRI and/or psychotherapy—slim pickings in the treatment department for so many complex issues. No wonder parents are exploring nutritional options, yoga, neurofeedback, and meditation.

BEYOND AMINO ACIDS

Because of Evie's fragile nature, I decided that trial and error with amino acid–based supplements was risky. Because she was already on Prozac, I did not want to target serotonin further with 5HTP and possibly increase it too much. Although sufficient serotonin is associated with a feeling of well-being, too much causes feelings of dissociation, a state of being unconnected from conscious or psychological functioning. In the medical world, this condition is called serotonin syndrome. Usually it's too much medication that gets you there, so piling 5HTP on top of the medication could theoretically be problematic.

Instead, I recommended a regimen using high-dose fish oil supplements, which could support general brain function with minimal potential for interfering with her ongoing medical treatment. Fish oil has not been studied much for the treatment of anxiety, but its use has been extensively followed in other neuropsychiatric disorders, including depression, so it required just a small cognitive stretch to see the possibilities.

USING FISH OIL TO BUILD A BETTER BRAIN

The way fish oil appears to work in the brain is complicated. Fish oil is a structural nutrient to some extent and incorporates into the membranes of the cell. The unique composition of the omega-3 fat, especially EPA (eicosapentaenoic acid), changes the properties and operating abilities of the membrane. This follows the basic architecture principle that function follows structure. Better materials, such as EPA, create a stronger, superior functioning structure, in this case the cell membrane. In architecture, a well-built house is more energy efficient, lasts longer, and is easier to live in (works better). The same can be said for a well-built cell.

The right kinds of fats improve the way the body's neurological system operates. The brain runs by changing chemical signals from neurotransmitters into electrical signals. Recall that the nerve cells send neurotransmitters across an itsy-bitsy space called a synapse. These chemical messengers have to be sent, received, and converted across the membranes quickly and fluidly with the least amount of interference. Inflammation and other conflicting messenger molecules create obstacles and traffic jams that make this process less efficient.

The omega-3 fatty acids, particularly EPA, provide the materials for the nervous system that reduce inflammation (and interference) the best and optimize the membrane's ability to send, receive, and convert signals in mood and cognitive disorders. DHA is also critical for brain development because it increases brain-derived neurotropic factor, a type of growth factor for the brain, but is not as useful for mood regulation.

The fish oil neuropsychiatric story started in 1998 when Dr. Joseph Hibbeln, a researcher at the National Institutes of Health, published his definitive study linking rates of major depression to fish consumption. Collecting data from all over the world, he shocked the medical community by finding a predictive relationship between how much fish different populations ate and their levels of depression. New Zealand, for example, where fish consumption is relatively low, had fifty times the depression rate of Japan, a country with a high rate of fish consumption. Bear in mind that association does not prove causation. Maybe the Japanese eat more fish because they are less depressed. Nonetheless, the caviar was out of the can, and newer studies have progressed toward proving an association. One study even compared the therapeutic effects of fluoxetine (Prozac) to fish oils. The amazing results found that fish oil worked as well as fluoxetine but that the combination of both treatments was superior to either of them alone. Evie was already on Prozac. Hmm.

THE RESEARCH ON OMEGA-3s

Evie did not have depression, so I decided to review the research on other neuropsychiatric disorders. Perhaps there would be enlightening or helpful information there.

Andrew Stoll, a Harvard researcher, found favorable results using omega-3 fats (mainly EPA) to treat bipolar disorder. In the classic 1999 study looking at the effectiveness of treating bipolar disorder with fish oil, the response from the group taking the fish oil was impressive. The flaw in the study was the placebo group. The placebo group has to be given the same number of similar-looking pills, and it was. The trouble arose because fish smells (and some fish oil pills do, too) and loads of pills are required to get to a therapeutic dose. One study participant who was getting the omega-3 was attacked by his cat whenever he took out the supplement, so he knew he was in the fish-taking group (or had a mean cat). Even without attack cats, most of the placebo group knew who they were by the second month and were not doing so well, so they dropped out.

Despite that design setback, the positive signs continue to pile up. There is evidence that omega-3 fats may help ADHD, Alzheimer's disease, schizophrenia, and other mood disorders. One study found a preliminary link between low levels of omega-3 fats and social anxiety disorder. The evidence is mounting, but the medical community is still taking a "let's wait and see" attitude.

While the medical community dukes out the fish oil question, Evie is getting older and more anxious. "Let's do more research" is an intellectual high ground that keeps the scientific community moving ahead, but is frustrating and plain old rotten for clinicians and patients suffering in the trenches. All the preliminary scientific evidence suggests that a high-potency EPA supplement could shift biochemical functioning in a direction that might help. So I thought that if Evie and her mother were game, why not try?

WHAT WE DID WITH EVIE

I put Evie on an omega-3 supplement that was 90 percent concentrated EPA. The total dose of EPA was 4 grams per day. She started with a smaller dose and worked up slowly to avoid the most common adverse side effects—gas and loose stools. The higher-quality fish oils are distilled and purified to remove heavy metal contaminants and reduce the chance

---

THEORIES ON HOW OMEGA-3 FATS WORK IN THE BRAIN
(WARNING: CONTAINS TECHNICAL INFORMATION)

Omega-3 fats are believed to positively shift cell mechanics and function in the following specific ways:

BIOCHEMICAL BENEFIT: Alters eicosanoid and cytokine pathways to reduce inflammation and improve mood.

ENGLISH TRANSLATION: Eicosanoids and cytokines are messenger or signaling molecules that operate all over the body. They send a massive amount of signals that regulate everything from the immune system to hormone secretion. Eicosanoids are a group of substances made from fats. Omega-3 fats like EPA tend to make anti-inflammatory ("good") eicosanoids, but other fats tend to make inflammatory or irritating eicosanoids. Some inflammation processes, like those associated with spraining your ankle or premenstrual swelling and weight gain you are aware of. Others, like the type that lay the foundation for heart disease and dementia, march along silently. Cytokines are made from protein and talk to the immune system. There are many different ones, and like eicosanoids, some create inflammation, but there are myriad other processes these chemicals regulate. Inflammation combined with the wrong cytokines may cause mood changes. EPA interferes with the production and mitigates the actions of other messenger molecules like cytokines.

BIOCHEMICAL BENEFIT: Reduction of abnormal signal transduction.

of fishy burps. Smelling like a dead fish was not going to improve her social life, and fish burps tend to reduce compliance, so using a high-quality product is absolutely critical. I threw in a multivitamin and mineral to optimize the use of the fatty acid supplement.

Evie was an advanced worrier, and I knew she was not going to become as calm as a Buddhist monk overnight, but I wanted to increase her coping capacity so she did not collapse under the weight of the daily aggravations of life. Her entire day's worth of stress tolerance could be shot by nine o'clock in the morning. Evie's level of worry was way beyond normal.

A more typical scenario was another preadolescent in my practice who barely had the tolerance to get through a school day but sweated

---

ENGLISH TRANSLATION: Signal transduction is how information travels across the space between nerve cells, is taken into the cell, and regulates its function.

BIOCHEMICAL BENEFIT: Improves cell membrane fluidity and neurotransmitter receptor function.

ENGLISH TRANSLATION: Fats are part of every cell wall. The omega-3 fats change the shape of structures embedded in the membranes, such as receptors for neurotransmitters. The superior structure of omega-3–rich membranes means the signal transduction of neurotransmitters, such as serotonin, can operate more smoothly and efficiently.

BIOCHEMICAL BENEFIT: Agonists of peroxisome proliferator-activated receptors (PPAR).

ENGLISH TRANSLATION: PPARs are genetic transcription factors. Genetic transcription factors are proteins that bind to specific DNA sections of a gene. This action tells the gene to transcribe that sequence of genetic information from DNA to messenger RNA. Messenger RNA takes the gene message to another part of the cell, where it is translated into protein production, and those proteins go and do the gene's bidding. *Agonist* means to produce an action or to help along. Put it all together, and fish oils support the actions of substances (PPARs) that help the genes function better. One of the jobs of genes is to oversee building and repair of the body. How omega-3 fats affect gene expression is not completely understood, but they appear to bring out the best of your brain's genetic potential. It all makes you wish you had paid attention in high school biology.

her way through. Sweet and compliant for her teachers, she was pinching her sisters and kicking her mother by four o'clock. When the mother demanded a conference to uncover what horrible situation had driven her child to extreme behaviors, she was met by baffled teachers. Perhaps, they hinted broadly, the mother was the one with anxiety issues. Anxiety has many different faces, depending on the severity, stressors, and temperament of the child. In both cases, I used EPA to increase capacity and function.

In about a month, Cheryl and Evie checked back in with me. "I think there is a difference, but I am not sure," Cheryl began. "It's subtle."

"Say more," I prompted. Jumping on the first piece of feedback tends not to go well. Parents are warming up, and the first thing they say can

CAN'T I JUST EAT MORE FISH?

You could and maybe should except for the pesky problem of mercury and PCB (polychlorinated biphenyl) contamination. The Environmental Protection Agency (the EPA you do not eat) and Food and Drug Administration (FDA) recommend that because of elevated mercury levels in fish, women of childbearing age, nursing mothers, and young children should eat *no more than* two servings per week of a variety of fish (for example, salmon, light tuna, shrimp, mackerel), and up to six ounces per week of albacore tuna. They earmark four species of fish to avoid entirely—golden bass (also known as tilefish), king mackerel, shark, and swordfish—larger, predatory fish that have higher levels of mercury. Meanwhile, the American Heart Association suggests consuming *at least* two servings per week of oily fish. Clinical data suggest that eating more fish significantly lowers cardiovascular mortality risk.

Studies have shown that PCBs and another environmental contaminant called dioxin may be carcinogenic. One study following women who ate fish with high PCB levels for years found that their babies had abnormal reflexes, general weakness, and more signs of depression. Their heads were also slightly smaller. Using PCB in manufacturing was banned in 1979, but it is still inadvertently produced as a by-product of manufacturing and leaches into the water, soil, and air. Fish caught in lakes and streams polluted by industrial waste or raised in farms fed by that same water can contain dangerous levels of PCBs.

Critics argue that PCBs are everywhere and that beef, chicken, pork, and cheese contain even higher levels than fish. You may have

reveal more about their own state of mind than what had actually happened since the last visit.

And the reality is that we, as parents, can be inaccurate observers of our own children, even though we know them best. The "knowing best" part may be the enemy of detached surveillance. We tend to define people early on and stick with our perceptions. "Mark always forgets where he puts his keys" or "Phyllis is always late." If Mark keeps track of his keys for an entire year then forgets them once, he is still the person who forgets his keys. If Phyllis breaks the late habit but gets caught in traffic, she is still considered a tardy person.

For better or worse, those labels can get stuck on children. Carlos, a nine-year-old boy who had four or five meltdowns per day, started

---

to avoid eating to avoid PCBs. The authors of a popular treatise on this issue published in the *Journal of the American Medical Association* assert, "The possible health risks of these low levels of PCBs and dioxins in fish are only a small fraction of the much better established health benefits of the omega-3 fatty acids. With the exception of some locally caught sport fish from contaminated inland waters, the levels of PCBs and dioxins in fish should not influence decisions about fish intake."

Nonetheless, do you really want to weigh the risk of getting cancer or shrinking the brain of your unborn child against reducing cardiovascular risk and improving the intelligence of that same unborn child every time you bite into a tuna sandwich? Add to that the problem of mercury contamination, sustainability, and the question of how much good omega-3 actually is in the fish.

Eating two 3–4-ounce servings per week of fish containing high amounts of EPA/DHA, like wild-caught salmon, provides a total of 2,800–3,500 milligrams of omega-3 fatty acids or an average of 400–500 milligrams per day. Take the average numbers with a grain of salt, because they vary greatly, depending on processing, time of year, type of fish, and how it was raised. A 6-ounce can of tuna may have as few as .9 gram of omega-3 oils or as many as 5.3 grams. That is a 500 percent difference.

You could literally drive yourself crazy. Best to eat a few servings per week of the small, safest fish (see "Sustainable Omega-3 Food Sources" on page 152), but for therapeutic purposes, take the extra omega-3s as a supplement. Stick with high-quality brands that have been purified and distilled.

NUTRITION DETECTIVE
PRINCIPLE #13

If you can't find any direct research about your issue, explore related conditions or studies.

Children are not studied as much as adults. The research is trickier, because the volunteer (the child) and the responsible party (the parent) are two different people. Research on kids involves twice the number of people to inform, keep track of, and demand compliance from. Furthermore, the standards are stricter because as a society we frown on using kids as guinea pigs. Who wants their child to be in the placebo group with a painful condition if there is a promising treatment?

Despite all this, there are ways to get clinical ideas from related research:

- First, look at research on other age groups and populations. There are many more studies on adults and neuropsychology, for example, than on children.

- Second, explore solutions for similar conditions. There is more research on depression and bipolar disorder than anxiety, for example, but they are all mood disorders.

- Third, look for similar symptoms. For example, let's say you cannot find anything useful for your child with juvenile rheumatoid arthritis. There may be useful research on other types of pain. Different types of pain can have similar inflammation processes, so maybe something there will help.

- Finally, be sure your theory, if acted upon, will do no harm.

taking fish oil at my suggestion. When I asked his mother how he was doing a month later, she swore there were no real changes. I asked her, "How many meltdowns is he having these days?" Her response? "One or two over the last week." From four or five a day to one or two a week is approximately an 80 percent improvement.

Luckily, I keep good notes. "Didn't you say he used to have four or five a day?" I pressed.

"Well, yes," his mother grumbled, "but he had one a few days ago, and I have zero tolerance left. One meltdown is too many."

Cheryl was in the same boat as Carlos's mother. Yes, Evie was getting off to school most days without incidents and she seemed generally happier, but she was still an above-average worrier. "I don't have much patience myself these days," Cheryl said upon reflection. "Do you think we could talk about my situation for a few minutes?" And we did.

Cheryl, Evie, and I agreed that the results were positive enough to continue without further adjustments and to give the program more time. Evie complied with taking the fish oils because she felt they helped and did not want to take more or other medicine. She managed better and better over time, although her anxious tendencies remained.

Is Your Child Overly Anxious?

If you have ever wondered if your child is a little more anxious than is strictly average, this questionnaire is for you.

☐ Does your child ask you the same question repeatedly?

☐ Is your child inflexible? For example, if plans change, does he have trouble adjusting to the new situation?

☐ Are you frequently reassuring your child because he expects something bad to happen?

☐ Does your youngster have trouble soothing himself?

☐ Does your child frequently use repetitive behaviors or rituals to calm down (such as talking to himself or holding certain objects)?

☐ Does your little one melt down easily if situations do not go his way?

☐ Would you describe your child as overly bossy or controlling?

☐ Are there too many tears or tantrums at your house given your child's age?

☐ Are you frequently asking yourself if your child's reaction is "normal"?

If you answer yes to three or more of these questions, your child may need help dealing with anxiety.

What to Do

1. The first step is to make an appointment with a pediatric mental health professional for an objective viewpoint. Perhaps some of the behaviors are developmentally within normal range and you only need some new parenting strategies to help your child manage better.

2. There are no easy answers for anxiety, but the most encouraging research suggests that a combination of corrective biochemistry and cognitive/behavioral therapy produces the most promising results. Nutritionally, the best biochemical tools available are a nutritious diet and a concentrated EPA supplement.

   Make sure your child is eating three meals per day and has a variety of fruit, vegetables, and whole grains, along with a good protein source, such as eggs, yogurt, nuts, beans, or fish, at each meal. Evie's mother had this step completed before we started with the therapeutic fish oil.

   Consider adding a high-quality, purified, 90 percent concentrated EPA fish oil supplement. Start with a smaller amount and work slowly up to the desired dose over a few weeks. Watch for loose stools or excessive fish burps. Consult an experienced health care professional for the exact dose for your child. In general, for children from ages three to six, the EPA dose will be between 1 and 3 grams. For ages seven and up, the dosage will be between 3 and 6 grams.

3. Combine improved chemistry with behavioral/cognitive therapy to help your child find effective coping techniques. When the brain is wired for worry, setting up new wires, which is what fish oil does, may not be enough. There have to be better nonworry messages sent through the new system to reset the operations. Repetitive experiences without anxiety are the foundation for permanent change. Practicing strengthens the new neurological pathways, leading to long-term learning.

4. Be patient. Learning to respond to situations in a new way takes months of practice. Expect some missteps on the road to mastery.

Learning and Behavior in Kids

CHAPTER 14

Two Cases of Chronic Ear Infections

F OR KIDS UNDER THE AGE OF THREE, ear infections are thought to be a common childhood nuisance. They hurt and they are annoying, but most toddlers seem to have them and, consequently, health care professionals wave them off as minor inconveniences. An antibiotic prescription here, an ear tube there, and eventually the infections are outgrown. End of story. Or is it?

Recurrent ear infections and fluid in the ears can be huge clues to health issues that can persist into adulthood. Although the youngster may outgrow inflamed ears, their underlying cause can often remain, stirring up other mischief. Let me tell you the stories of two kids who both had chronic ear infections. One was treated early, and the other "outgrew" the infections and came to see me for something else—or so his parents thought.

EMILY'S ACHING EARS

W hen I met Emily, she was two years old. She'd gotten her first ear infection (known in medical parlance as otitis media) soon after she turned six months old, and got two or three more before turning one. At that point she had a few healthy months, then got another two or three ear infections over the next six months. Her doctor recommended ear tube placement to ease her discomfort, but Emily's parents (she had two mothers) looked at their tiny toddler and decided to wait. Maybe Emily would outgrow the nasty infections, as many children do they reasoned.

But the cycle continued. Emily would be fine for a couple of months, and then she'd have two or three more ear infections, reigniting the ear tube discussion. As the ear infection number approached double digits, Emily's parents decided they could watch and wait no longer. They would either have to get tubes or do something else to break the vicious cycle.

> For unknown reasons, the number of children with developmental challenges is rising at an alarming rate, and in my experience, too many of them have a history of chronic ear infections.

By the time I was introduced to Emily, her worried moms had almost talked themselves into putting Emily through ear tube surgery. Emily's pediatrician was understanding about their concerns and had been willing to wait. But now he was beginning to push for surgery. The ear infections were frequent enough that Emily's language development seemed to be affected, adding a new brick to the worry pile. Emily was making sounds, but she was not speaking as clearly or as fluently as her peers. The pediatrician had assured her moms that Emily was developing normally so far, but everyone was starting to get nervous.

Emily's parents were right to be concerned about frequent ear infections and long-term development. Chronic ear infections and/or ear fluid have long been associated with speech delays. The common wisdom is that most children overcome speech impediments once the ear infections clear up, but I am not comfortable with this thinking. For unknown reasons, the number of children with developmental challenges is rising at an alarming rate, and in my experience, too many of them have a history of chronic ear infections.

AUDITORY DEVELOPMENT

A child may be born with ears, but it takes several years for her to learn to fully use them. The newborn baby experiences the world as a cacophony of noise that must be sorted and assigned meaning. After many exposures to a certain high-pitched string of sounds, baby starts associating this melody with the arrival of lunch and an important soothing figure: mom. Over time the infant learns to pinpoint sound and look toward the approaching figure. Recognizing it, she smiles. She learns which sounds are significant and which ones should be ignored. By age one, the baby notices she gets good feedback if she imitates some of these pleasant noises, and the beginnings of language are born.

This is a very stripped-down version of auditory processing development. The full version is complex and evolves sequentially over several years. Now what happens if the wee one is trying to learn to use her ears but they are frequently full of fluid or infected? The sounds are distorted and harder to read. During the critical developmental milestone period for auditory processing (birth to age three), if her ears are not operating properly, she will not learn how to listen with them effectively. By age four or five, the ears may be infection-free, but significant periods of training time were missed. Now the child can hear sounds but has not assigned proper meaning to them. What to pay attention to and what to screen out are not obvious to children who spent much of their auditory training period with clogged ears. As a result, these children cannot listen as well or imitate sounds or words as clearly as their peers, and their overall language development may be slowed.

Because babies have tiny heads, are lying down most of the time, and cannot blow their noses, any mucus that forms tends to drip back into the ear canals. (And where there's mucus, there's a growth opportunity for organisms that cause infections.) The ear canals, sinuses, and back of the throat are all connected through a series of tubes. That is why sometimes when you blow your nose, your ears pop.

Emily's ear infections had to be stopped—that was clearly the first order of business. But I had to figure out their cause.

I delved into her history and learned from her moms that Emily had always been a pale, fussy kid. Her first ear infection was diagnosed about a month after she stopped nursing and started on a milk-based formula. Then when she turned one, formula was traded in for whole milk and yogurt, both of which Emily loved. When I met Emily, her entire diet consisted of milk, yogurt, pizza, pasta with cheese, bread, and fruit.

This is a story I hear over and over again; ear infections starting right after a baby is weaned from the breast or switched from formula to regular milk. Dr. Talal Nsouli, an ear, nose, and throat specialist in the Washington, D.C., area, must have heard similar stories, because in 1994 he published a study that looked at chronic ear infections and their relationship to food intolerance. He reported that about 90 percent of kids with recurring ear infections or ear fluid had positive markers for food allergies and that when those foods were removed from the diet, the ear infections/fluid went away. When the foods were reintroduced, the infections came back. The number one problem food was milk. The specific irritant is milk protein (casein). Soy, wheat, and eggs were the other identified reactors in the children studied.

Given this research and Emily's strong preference for dairy foods, as well as the timing of her illnesses (they started after the introduction of milk-based formula and then whole milk), cow's milk protein (casein) seemed like the most obvious potential irritant.

So now I had several clues:

- frequent ear infections (meaning more than three in total before age four)

- first onset after switching to milk-based formula

- increased infection frequency after moving from formula (which contains predigested milk) to whole milk

- speech delays

I shared my suspicions with Emily's parents. Despite their anxiety that she would not get enough protein because almost all the protein in her diet came from dairy-based foods, we took Emily off all foods containing significant amounts of casein, including milk, ice cream, yogurt, and cheese. She could still have small amounts of dairy products baked into food, such as milk used to make bread or milk fat–derived foods (like butter). "Is she going to starve?" one of her moms asked, looking for reassurance.

All that was left in Emily's diet was bread, pasta, and fruit. There was not enough protein, and if she did not eat more to fill in for the foods we were removing, there would not be enough calories. I was hoping for the appearance of a surprising but common occurrence—the suddenly-will-eat-other-foods-when-dairy-is-removed phenomenon—and explained this possibility to her moms. I also suggested the addition of a multivitamin/mineral and a calcium supplement.

After a few days of very little eating and very much fussing, Emily tentatively started trying some new foods, including salmon and chicken. Within a few weeks, her fussiness all but disappeared. Most important, the ear infections stopped and did not recur. Yes, the response was practically a miracle, and for this reason, I hesitated to include this case in this book. I don't want parents to think that removing dairy products from the diet always miraculously erases ear infections (or cures picky eating). Sometimes other foods need to be removed also, and occasionally there are other, nonnutritional issues. On the other hand, I have had so many similar cases that I am shocked and disturbed that this information is not better known. The misery and developmental problems that could be avoided by applying this simple strategy are enormous.

Emily continued to develop normally, and her early minor speech delays disappeared. Her ear infection trend had been curtailed early enough that she quickly got back on track. Emily was happier and healthier, and all was well.

Fortunately, because Emily's situation was addressed early, a simple solution remedied a painful and potentially damaging childhood problem. As you'll see, not all cases are so miraculous.

BEHIND DANIEL'S ADHD

I met eleven-year-old Daniel after he'd had an extensive neuropsycho-logical evaluation, which his teachers had recommended because he had trouble following directions, paying attention, and turning in assignments on time. The Intelligence Quotient (IQ) part of the extensive and expensive test indicated that Daniel was a closet rocket scientist. His parents were not shocked at how high his IQ was, but wondered whether

THE SUDDENLY-WILL-EAT-OTHER-FOODS-WHEN-DAIRY-IS-REMOVED PHENOMENON

For unknown reasons, people often crave foods to which they are sensitive. But there are several theories for why we yearn for reactive foods. They all sound like something you would read about in a science fiction book but are based on known biological principles. Here are the best two to date (they are not mutually exclusive—they can operate simultaneously):

THEORY ONE relates specifically to why gluten and casein proteins can cause an addiction response: Gluten and casein proteins are complicated, and some individuals may be short on an enzyme needed to break them down completely. The result of this impeded digestive process is that the proteins turn into an unusual, incompletely processed molecule with a structure similar to morphine. In the nervous system, the receptor sites for endorphins (natural painkillers) mistakenly accept the

alien compound, thereby activating a painkilling but also addictive neurological response. This feels mighty good, and the body wishes to repeat the experience as often as possible. The conscious mind may not know what happened, but the body knows. Thus, milk- and/or wheat-based foods are highly desired. Even with the painkilling response, people can still experience discomfort, because higher levels of endorphins cannot override all levels and sources of pain any more than drugs can erase all misery.

THEORY TWO: Some scientists suspect that the body gets addicted to the chemical messengers triggered by allergic reactions. Histamine and cortisol (a relative of adrenaline) are typically released during classic allergy reactions, but who knows what fun, problematic messenger molecules could be released by other types of sensitivities? There is a whole complex chemistry surrounding messenger molecules, among them cytokines. Cytokines can cause depression, raise body temperature, or increase inflammation. Scientists

he could get into rocket-scientist school if he never turned in any home-work. "What good is a stellar IQ if he flunks out of middle school?" his father deadpanned.

IQ is a measure of potential for learning, not performance. A high number denotes a superior capacity for assimilating knowledge, but is not a measure of mastery. Daniel's parents were well aware of the differ-ence between tested IQ and performance IQ. They were not comforted

have become very interested in the many complex ways cytokines modulate responses to allergens, illness, mood, and myriad other processes, including addiction. Nobody yet knows how they set up an environment to cause addiction, but they are suspected to have a critical role. They come and go quickly and are hard to study, so we do not know half of what they are up to, but they are always up to something.

THE BOTTOM LINE IS THIS: When the irritating food is eliminated from the diet, after a short adjustment period, some children snap out of their dietary daze and are suddenly more open to new food experiences. Although a parent cannot depend on this phenomenon, it may be worth removing the irritant first to see what, if anything, happens. Your child might "suddenly" be more amenable to new foods. If not, you can always pull out the E.A.T. program (see page 52) or consider other feeding interventions.

One mother told me that her daughter, a fussy eater, would wake up crabby and demand chocolate milk. Thinking milk was healthy, she would hand over a cupful only to watch her toddler guzzle it like a frat boy and transform in front of her eyes into a sweet child. "It was kind of creepy," she reported. "It was almost like she was addicted to it and I had given her a hit." The mom decided to take dairy products out of her child's diet for a while to see if her daughter would become less persnickety about food. She did, and no other behavioral interventions were necessary.

The problem with attempting behavioral interventions if the child is "addicted" to a food is that sometimes they don't work. Like an addict, the child will often prefer not to eat at all if not given her drug of choice or she just asks for the irritant over and over. Just like you cannot successfully work on a marriage problem if one of the parties is a drug addict until the substance abuse is resolved, you cannot work on a feeding issue until the addictive food is removed. Otherwise, the child is at the mercy of her own internal neurochemicals and will not be amenable to help.

by his high IQ score. Daniel was not living up to his potential, and as he was getting older and expectations increased, the situation was getting worse.

The most common explanation for a large testing versus performance gap is ADHD. The psychologist who conducted the testing concluded that Daniel probably had a form of ADHD, and as a result introduced the idea of treating him with medicines. But his parents were not at all comfortable with this line of thinking or treatment.

And they were right to be suspicious.

Before launching into my own very strong bias against the quickness to diagnose ADHD, I tried to calm Daniel's parents by first asking them some questions about their son's early years.

I was not surprised to learn that he had suffered from multiple ear infections as a baby and as a toddler. The ear infections were long gone, but now Daniel was prone to sinus infections, often had a stuffy nose and eczema, and suffered from frequent environmental allergies (including reactions to cats, pollen, and ragweed). He was already on year-round allergy medicine, which is one of the reasons his mother was not happy about putting him on more medicine for ADHD. Furthermore, she was worried that the ADHD medicine would change or flatten out Daniel's personality.

Here are the clues so far:

- a history of frequent ear infections
- year-round allergies
- capacity versus performance gap

The next clue? When I asked about his diet, I learned that like many preteens, his diet was heavy on waffles and sandwiches and light on fruits and vegetables. He needed more string beans and less string cheese, but luckily he was not drinking much soda and was not a big sweets eater. Then his mom mentioned almost proudly that Daniel loved milk and drank a few glasses every day. "Thank God he gets all that protein and calcium," she said.

But to me, this preference for dairy was a clue, given his frequent congestion, allergies, and history of ear infections. All of these conditions can involve mucus, and mucus can form in response to irritation.

As babies get bigger heads (and develop wider ear canals), spend more time upright, and can better control their snot (i.e., begin to blow their noses), fluid does not build up behind their eardrums as much. Mucus gets stuck in other places in the nasal passages and throat labyrinth, and where the mucus goes, infection follows. The goo that drips down the back of the throat (or into the ear canals) is the perfect growing medium for whatever germs are floating around home, day care, or preschool. Bacteria need warmth, dampness (or something to stick to), nutrients to eat, and time to grow. A baby's ear canal or child's sinus cavity is just perfect. The more fluid there is and the longer it sits in a 98-degree passage, the better for breeding infection. Attracting germs is never a problem, because they are everywhere.

If whatever was causing your child's ear infections is still a factor in his life, the symptoms and/or irritation may have moved out of his ears and into another part of his body.

I thought more about Daniel's other symptoms:

- With growth and development, Daniel's vulnerable spot for bug colonization could have moved from his ear passages to his sinuses.

- He also had environmental allergies. When children continue to consume irritants, the constant assault to the immune system can make them more reactive to other allergens.

My emerging theory was that Daniel had a long-standing sensitivity to dairy products. As an infant, the reaction manifested as ear infections, but as he continued guzzling milk, the infection place shifted to his sinuses. And because he was already reacting to dairy, he was more reactive to environmental agents and had developed pollen and other outdoor allergies.

Daniel's parents were not surprised by my suggestion to stop giving him dairy products. As is often the case, they were suspicious about dairy products themselves, but because they could not get confirmation from a medical professional, they had never followed up with an elimination trial. We all agreed to take dairy products out of Daniel's diet for six weeks.

His response? Daniel's sinuses improved dramatically, and he was able to discontinue his year-round allergy medicine. He still needed to take allergy medicine for a few months in the spring when tree-pollen

EAR INFECTIONS AND AUTISM

As the number of children receiving a diagnosis of autism spectrum disorders (ASD) soars, parents and scientists are looking for controllable risk factors. ASD is a set of developmental disorders characterized by communication deficits, repetitive impaired patterns of behavior, and social interaction impairment. Nobody knows what causes autism, and everyone would be happy if ear infections were the culprit, because then we could fix this horrible epidemic. Although ear infections by themselves do not cause autism, many children with autism also have a history of frequent ear infections and an intolerance of dairy.

Researchers have noted that children with autism have more ear infections than neurotypical children. One study found that children with autism had ten times more ear infections during their first three years than typical kids. The lower-functioning children on the spectrum had earlier onset of ear infections compared with the higher-functioning children. Although more ear infections occurring together with autism does not mean one causes

the other, factors that make a child more susceptible to ear infections may also make him more vulnerable to neurological issues.

One factor may be related to overall immune weaknesses. Dr. Marie Bristol-Power, a scientist at the National Institute of Child Health and Human Development, presented mounting evidence of immune dysfunction in autism in a 2001 meeting of the Institute of Medicine. She was quoting the seminal work of the late Dr. Reed Warren, which found a number of immune deficiencies in children with autism. The relationship between the immune problems and neurological development is now well known, although nobody knows exactly what that relationship is. What we do know is that the immune system talks to the neurological system using our old friends the messenger molecules called cytokines. Neurotransmitters and other neuropeptides also send messages back and forth.

These messages from the immune system can and do affect neurodevelopment and behavior, especially during vulnerable periods. The time between birth and three is one of those vulnerable periods for

counts were high, and he took it if he stayed overnight somewhere with cats, but overall he felt much healthier. His ability to pay attention also improved, helping his school performance.

However, because his auditory processing had been impeded as a young child, removing the dairy irritant at age eleven did not retroactively correct his listening abilities. Daniel still did not fully know how to use

development, and this is typically when ear infections strike. If a child is sick a lot during this period, could this tip the scales toward autism?

Perhaps the illnesses themselves would not cause autism, but the stress of them added to other unknown genetic factors and environmental stressors might cause some children to suffer neurologically who otherwise would not. ASD involves many causative factors we do not understand and cannot control, but if pressure can be taken off the nervous system by preventing ear infections, I say let's do it.

A diet eliminating potential irritants seems like a small, prudent step if it would help reduce risk factors for this devastating condition. These days, many doctors and therapists helping parents whose children have autism are recommending a gluten-free, casein-free diet and witnessing an increase in functioning.

Complicating the possible ear infection–autism connection is the usual antibiotic treatment for ear infections. Dr. Joan Fallon, a chiropractor from New York, published a paper in 2005 implicating the antibiotic Augmentin as an ASD causative factor. She also noted the higher incidence of ear infections in children with ASD, observing that those children received an average of twelve courses of antibiotics. Augmentin is an effective treatment for ear infections, especially those resistant to amoxicillin, an older, simpler antibiotic. The more ear infections, the higher the chance of a child receiving a broader-spectrum antibiotic such as Augmentin. Fallon postulated that high-risk children could become autistic from exposure to the potent neurotoxin ammonia. Augmentin is manufactured using a fermentation process that involves urea/ammonia.

In the end, the noted relationship between ear infections and autism raises more questions than it answers. Are ear infections a cause or effect of other factors contributing to autism? Is the problem the ear infections themselves affecting auditory processing, their treatment with antibiotics, underlying immune dysfunction, and/or food intolerance (of which ear infections are one symptom)? While we are grappling to find answers to these questions, what we do know is that ear infections should be taken seriously when they occur.

his ears. He would "forget" multistep directions and was still too distracted at school. His parents had to pursue additional corrective therapy to help improve his auditory processing. There are a number of programs now available to enhance and to help further auditory development, including the Tomatis Program, Earobics, The Listening Program–Music-Based Auditory Stimulation, Samonas Auditory Training programs, and Fast ForWord, to name a few. These programs are usually offered by occupational, speech, or educational therapists. After completing one of the above programs, one twelve-year-old commented, "Now I can actually hear myself think."

If your son or daughter needs help with auditory processing, you may have to consult with several speech and occupational therapists to find a program that is right for your child. It is an evolving field of exploration and has not hit the mainstream yet. The important take-away is this: Just because you stop sitting on tacks does not mean you are completely healed. Post-tack-sitting corrective measures may be necessary to clean up the damage.

So what would have happened if Daniel's parents had pursued the ADHD diagnosis and treated his distraction and inability to focus with medicine? Medication would have made Daniel sit in his seat better, but it would not have helped him learn how to use his brain. A developmental approach goes back and walks him through what he missed the first time. Removing the dairy and getting the right therapy put Daniel back on track. He struggled over the next several years but slowly started to master

NUTRITION DETECTIVE PRINCIPLE #14

Timing is everything.

When it comes to identifying the clues of your child's health situation, it's important to consider timing. What was happening around the time the problem started? For example, many children begin having ear infections at twelve months when they are traditionally switched from infant formula, which is easier to digest, to whole milk. Because we now know ear fluid buildup and infections are highly associated with food intolerance, thinking about whether or not there were dietary or formula changes at the time of the onset of the infections may help you narrow down the likely culprit.

his meandering mind. Although this approach took longer and involved more of his input than medicine would have, everyone was pleased with the results.

ARE FREQUENT EAR INFECTIONS AN EARLY RISK FACTOR FOR LATER ADHD?

In a word, yes. Of course, we need decades more of studies to prove it with absolute certainty. Nonetheless, the connections are logical.

ADHD is not so much a disease as a cluster of nonspecific symptoms lacking clear causation. The National Institute of Mental Health describes ADHD as "one of the most common childhood disorders and can continue through adolescence and adulthood. Symptoms include difficulty staying focused and paying attention, difficulty controlling behavior, and hyperactivity (over-activity)."

The general nature of the condition does beg the question: What would make a child distracted? One likely suspect is poor auditory processing development. Studies following children with a history of frequent ear infections found they tended to be more distracted all the way through high school than children who didn't have early ear troubles. Today, distracted adolescents are apt to be diagnosed with ADHD, raising disturbing questions about the relationship of early ear infections to later attention issues.

People with a well-developed auditory processing system can prioritize information coming in through their ears. For example, they can decide to listen to the teacher giving out the homework assignment and not pay attention to Nicky tapping his pencil. When the processing is poor, all of that information has the same priority, so it sticks randomly. A child may not hear the homework assignment because he is distracted by his friend who is whacking his pencil against the desk.

Auditory processing has a huge effect on executive functioning. If the science teacher says, "Take out a piece of lined paper, fold it lengthwise, and put your name on the top right-hand corner," you can do that after hearing it once. The child whose auditory development went astray takes out the lined paper and "forgets" what else he is supposed to do.

These are the symptoms of ADHD, but when the medical history includes long stretches of ear infections or fluid in the ear, I call it post-traumatic ear infection syndrome (PEIS) because I believe much of the distractibility comes from a poorly functioning auditory system. Not all ADHD is related to PEIS. But the specific distinction, when relevant, helps identify a treatable cause, whereas ADHD only describes the symptoms.

Are Past or Present Ear Infections an Issue for Your Child?

Ear infections are very common, so it's easy to dismiss their potentially damaging effect. These questions will help you determine if any current ear infections signal danger or if there might be a residual effect from past occurrences in your child's life.

- ☐ Did your child have more than three ear infections before the age of three?

- ☐ Does she have a history of a lot of fluid in her ears?

- ☐ Were ear infections or ear fluid found at well-baby visits with the pediatrician?

- ☐ Does your child have a high pain threshold?

- ☐ Does your child tend to pull or dig in her ears a lot?

- ☐ Have you noticed that your child talks rather loudly?

- ☐ Is your child hard to understand when she talks or has she been diagnosed with articulation issues?

- ☐ Does your child have trouble following two- and three-step directions?

- ☐ Is or was your child's speech delayed?

- ☐ Has your child with a history of frequent early ear infections gotten a diagnosis of Attention Deficit Disorder (ADD) or ADHD?

□ Is your child easily distracted or inattentive?

If you answered yes to three or more of the above questions, ear infections are a present or residual significant issue for your child and may be the result of her consuming an irritant.

What to Do

1. Try an elimination diet. The following four foods are most associated with ear infections: dairy products, wheat, soy, and eggs. Before eliminating all of these foods from the diet, consider taking dairy products and soy out first. This change alone is often sufficient to reduce or stop infections.

2. Have your child take a probiotic. Found in the refrigerator section of health food stores, probiotics balance the digestive tract and reduce allergic tendencies. (For more on probiotics, see page 126.) Ear infections are treated with antibiotics, which kill both good and bad bacteria, leaving many children short on the good guys. It may take some trial and error to find the right probiotic for your individual situation. Some are too strong and will increase gas and irritability; others are not potent enough. If the probiotic causes side effects and symptoms are not alleviated in a few days, reduce the dose, change brands, or consult with a health care professional familiar with using probiotics therapeutically.

3. Have your child's auditory processing skills evaluated. If your distracted child has a history of ear infections, her auditory processing abilities may have been affected. Auditory processing abilities can be determined by educational assessment. Once the problem areas have been identified, a plan can be made to address them.

   Ear infections and their nasty remnant, PEIS, are very common and mostly preventable. An ounce of prevention is worth years of distraction.

CHAPTER 15

The Tales of Chuck and Dale

O VER THE PAST FEW YEARS, we've been hearing and reading more and more about the benefits of "eating organic," especially for pregnant women and our children. According to the Organic Trade Association, Americans spent $28 billion on organic food in 2008, which is an increase of almost $27 billion from 1990 and indicates a dramatic shift in consumers' belief in organic foods as a healthier alternative to conventionally grown or raised foods. And despite these tough economic times, demand is projected to increase even further.

Is it important to choose organic food for growing children? How bad can a few sprayed grapes and apples really be? And if they are harmful, why isn't the Food and Drug Administration or Environmental Protection Agency (EPA) controlling the danger? The answers are simple: yes, pretty bad, and it's complicated.

A number of new studies have shown that the pesticides used to grow nonorganic foods damage the still-developing nervous and immune systems of children (details on this a little later). What complicates the situation is that, for the most part, the connections between eating chemically or genetically altered food and health problems are vague and tenuous. But every once in a while you can see a clear correlation, as in the stories of Chuck and Dale.

CHUCK AND HIS STRAWBERRIES

I have known Chuck since he was three. When I met him, he had recently received a diagnosis of autism and was nonverbal. His mother, Rosita, is optimistic, devoted, and a fireball. She and her family have pursued alternative treatments for autism, and Chuck adheres to a complex regimen of nutritional supplements and a strict elimination diet. Now, more than ten years later, with the help of a dedicated team of therapists, a set of forward-thinking doctors, diet intervention, and nutritional supplements, Chuck has made tremendous progress, showing slow but steady improvement.

When Chuck's autism was first diagnosed, he was extremely irritable and constantly agitated. But under his mother's regimen, he became calmer, learning to communicate verbally and to interact with his peers. Now at thirteen, Chuck was still on the autistic spectrum, but he was doing well in his special education program and could hold a basic conversation. For ten years, Rosita had kept him on a strict diet, avoiding foods containing not only gluten and casein but also sugar and a few other foods that his allergist found to be a problem. Yes, it meant avoiding a lot of foods, but Rosita insisted that sugar and the other eliminated foods made Chuck irritable when he ate them. He ate meats, vegetables, some nuts, seeds, whole grains, and a limited amount of fruit. It was a healthy diet most of us can only aspire to.

However, recently Chuck had begun to pay more attention to the array of foods that his peers were eating, and he wanted to expand his repertoire. Over the years Rosita had tried to add some of the eliminated foods, but she always noticed an immediate deterioration in Chuck's behavior or ability to focus if, for example, he had ice cream or pasta. "Is there anything else he can eat?" she asked me.

Because I had known Chuck for more than a decade, I approached his mother's dilemma already armed with a lot of information about him, so I skipped my usual clue-finding steps. My thinking was that because Chuck had been stable for so long, he should at least be able to handle more fruit. And Chuck loved the proposition!

We decided to start by adding strawberries because they are a low-allergen food and were in season. The berries were a hit—Chuck loved them and was extremely happy about his new treat.

But a few days later, I received a frantic call from Rosita, who said Chuck had a rash developing all over his face. Disappointed, she stopped buying strawberries and reported the trial a failure. They were both understandably frustrated, because there had been no reason to think Chuck would react, which is why I had recommended them.

In Chuck's case, the clues we had were pretty straightforward:

- very clean, strict diet most of his life
- already reactive or allergic to many foods
- developmental delays making him potentially more neurologically or immunologically sensitive
- appearance of rash shortly after consuming the trial food

Because we had set up a controlled trial, it did not take Stephen Hawking to deduce that strawberries caused the rash. What we did not know was whether Chuck's reaction was just another allergy or something else was going on.

Rosita and I did not want to give up on expanding Chuck's diet, nor did she wish to drag her son back to the allergist for yet another set of tests. We discussed waiting for the rash to clear and then starting another trial with a new fruit when I remembered an article I had read on pesticide residues.

According to the Environmental Working Group (www.ewg.org), strawberries have among the highest levels of pesticide residue of all the produce on the market. Environmental Working Group is a Washington, D.C.–based nonprofit group that supports environmental research, advocates on Capitol Hill for health protection policies, and disseminates information about the environment and public health. Because strawberries are very porous, they absorb whatever is sprayed on them. Unlike bananas, which can be peeled, or hard-skin fruit that can be scrubbed, all you can do with strawberries is rinse them off and hope for the best. The fruit itself may not be very reactive, but I knew the pesticides used to grow them could be. Before moving on to a new fruit, I suggested that Rosita try organic strawberries after the rash resolved.

THE POISON ON OUR PLANTS

The good news is that Chuck is now eating as many strawberries as he can hold without any problem, as long as they are organic. The bad news is that although figuring out the cause of Chuck's reaction was not particularly difficult, most cases of pesticide reactions are not nearly this clear. How many children are on such a strict and regulated diet that you can so easily isolate the problem food? Not many. If a child is having a direct reaction to something sprayed on his food, the symptoms usually look like some type of allergic reaction. There can be rashes, stomachaches, throat itching, or crankiness. But should you be concerned if there are no direct reactions? Yes, because not getting sick immediately is too low a standard to set for food safety. We don't know enough about what will happen down the line. Current research has shown significant ties of pesticides to triggering developmental delays. But since we cannot predict all the small or large effects caused by these poisons, I suggest we err on the side of caution.

Pesticides, like so many inventions, were developed by accident. Nobody set out specifically to find better ways to kill bugs on crops. Instead, scientists were looking for better ways to kill people, specifically our enemies during World War II. Chemistry had advanced enough for our intrepid researchers to develop effective nerve poisons, and they did so in quantity.

Luckily, the war ended before we could use all of the poison we had developed. Consequently, by the end of the 1940s, we had warehouses full

ARE ORGANIC FOODS MORE NUTRITIOUS?

Yes. They have to be by definition. To successfully raise food organically, the plants have to be healthier to resist pests, meaning the soil has to contain higher levels of nutrients. The plants take in these nutrients. The second reason is that nutrients, like vitamin C, are created within a plant when a plant's internal defense mechanisms are triggered by fighting a pest. We think of pesticides as being bad because of the chemical makeup of synthetic commercial pesticides, but natural pest deterrents are indigenous to the plant, and some are nutrients for us.

Fascinating research elucidating the mechanisms of how all this works is piling up. There are also many studies directly comparing the nutrient content of organic versus conventionally raised food. The Organic Center (TOC), a nonprofit organization (www.organic-center.org) dedicated to generating credible, peer-reviewed scientific information about organic products, has amassed a robust amount of data. TOC reviewed ninety-seven studies and concluded that the nutrient levels of organic foods, on average, were 25 percent higher than the same conventionally raised items. Some individual studies have found more vitamin C in organic oranges, more lycopene (a cancer-preventing antioxidant) in organic tomatoes, and more cancer-fighting antioxidants in organic corn, blackberries, and strawberries.

Naysayers argue that there is not enough research, organic food is too expensive, and it is not practical for feeding the masses. The financial aspects of how to raise safe food for hundreds of millions of people are way beyond my expertise, but I can tell you it is more nutritious.

---

of the stuff. Rather than waste in peacetime everything they created, the chemists reconfigured the compounds in much lower doses so they could be used to kill insects and other pests. (*Pesticide* is a general term used to refer to any substance, biological agent, or device used to kill any type of rodent, microbe, or pathogens. *Insecticides* specifically target insects.) But these commercial insecticides and pesticides were originally meant as human-icides and are still toxic to people. However, because the doses are so small, it is difficult to clearly associate exposure to a specific compound with resulting symptoms.

Organophosphates, one of the most common types of insecticides, work by inhibiting cholinesterase in the nervous system. Cholinesterase is an enzyme that controls the neurotransmitter acetylcholine, which operates in the spaces between the nerve cells. (For more on how neurotransmitters work, see page 211.) By disrupting acetylcholine, high exposure to organophosphates interferes with the part of the nervous system that runs the muscles. The result is muscle twitching and depressed motor control, including breathing. Imagine the teenage monster movie where the cute girl or doomed best friend gets bitten by the alien-possessed boyfriend, starts twitching, curls up in a fetal position, and expires, and you get the general idea.

Of course, this does not happen if you eat, say, a conventionally raised peach without washing it. Usually what happens is absolutely nothing other than you really enjoy it—or perhaps find it a little mealy, if it's from a bad crop. And this is exactly the problem. Most of us can handle small amounts of toxins without a noticeable ill effect, but at some unknown point of concentration (and it's likely different for everyone), these poisons start causing subtle sensory and behavior disturbances, lack of coordination, and depressed motor function.

Might pesticide consumption account for why so many children have attention, health, and other behavioral issues? It is impossible to say or prove, but emerging studies are raising disturbing questions. The medical journal *Pediatrics* recently published a study looking at a link between attention-deficit hyperactivity disorder (ADHD) and exposure to organophosphate pesticides. Pesticides break down into chemicals that scientists can measure in the urine. Studying urine samples from more than a thousand children, they found that higher pesticide residues increased the chances of the child having ADHD. A California Department of Public Health study

> Most of us can handle small amounts of toxins without a noticeable ill effect, but at some unknown point of concentration, these poisons start causing subtle sensory and behavior disturbances, lack of coordination, and depressed motor function.

published in the journal *Environmental Health Perspectives* found that women living near fields sprayed with organochlorine pesticides (a close relative of organophosphorus pesticides) were more likely to give birth to children with autism spectrum disorders. Another study in that journal found that children who substituted organic fruits and vegetables for their conventionally grown counterparts had lower amounts of organophosphorus pesticides in their urine.

In 2000, a National Academy of Sciences study "suggested that one out of four developmental and behavioral problems in children may be linked to genetic and environmental factors including exposure to lead, mercury, and organophosphate pesticides." Then there are the studies that found a statistical increase in cancer risk related to amount and type of pesticide exposure. Taken all together, it is enough to make any parent nervous. It also raises the question of why we aren't doing more as a country to reduce pesticide use or at least understand the risks better.

According to Dr. Michael Firestone, a senior scientist and expert on children's environmental health at the EPA, we are trying. Since 2000, the EPA in conjunction with the National Institute of Environmental Health Services has jointly funded several children's research centers to look at the effect of environmental issues on children's health. A large-scale national children's study, conducted by the National Institutes of Health and other organizations, looking at pesticides and hormone disruptors is also in the planning stages, but these projects are extremely complicated and expensive. As Dr. Firestone tactfully explains, "You cannot do direct testing on children." In other words, you cannot dose kids up with a particular pesticide and see if they get mean or stop reading or fall ill.

Instead, you can use epidemiological data, look for associations, and calculate percentage risk. Epidemiological data is information gathered from studying patterns of sickness and health in specific populations. It is used by public health officials to identify risk factors and causes of disease so that effective prevention and treatment strategies can be developed. Much epidemiological data about pesticide use is amassed because of the misfortune of people who have been accidentally acutely poisoned. Underpaid migrant farmers or factory workers are often the unwitting subjects of these studies. Although undoubtedly many of them have gotten sick from pesticide exposure, this observation does not help as much as you might think. Most people are not handling pesticides all day, so applying the disturbing findings to a more general population does not work. We have very little information about what smaller exposures to various poisons do over a long period of time.

For example, one very disturbing epidemiological study tested the blood from the umbilical cords of newborn babies from five states

PESTICIDE EFFECTS AT A GLANCE

Here's a quick roundup of some of the proven harmful effects that exposure to pesticides can have on us humans:

- low birth weight and birth defects
- interference with child development and cognitive ability
- neurological problems
- disruption of hormone function
- a variety of cancers, including leukemia, kidney cancer, brain cancer, and non-Hodgkin's lymphoma

Children and fetuses suffer more of these effects from pesticides than adults do because their bodily systems are still developing and they are smaller, so the concentrations are higher. Additionally, children are much less able than adults to detoxify most pesticides. Pesticide effects in the unborn and in infants can have lifelong consequences. The neurological or behavioral problems resulting from early pesticide exposure continue through puberty, as the reproductive system, nervous system, and brain grow, incorporating the effects of the chemicals. Also worth noting is the fact that farm workers suffer more than their share of bad pesticide effects, as well as the birds, beneficial insects, and other wild critters that are unwittingly in harm's way.

Pesticide exposure can occur through means other than food intake. Farm workers and home gardeners can handle it and absorb some through the skin, for example, or you can breathe it in if you or your neighbor is spraying it. Nonetheless, research shows that reducing pesticide consumption via food has an immediate observable effect on body-burden levels of pesticides. So, when you're in the produce aisle, pick organic when you can, and when you can't, try to avoid foods with high pesticide residues, substituting those with low pesticide residues (see the chart on page 257).

between December 2007 and June 2008. The researchers were looking for the presence of industrial chemicals, pesticides, and pollutants. The result found 232 potentially toxic chemicals already in their blood the day they were born. Frightening to be sure, but what does it mean? If two of those children develop autism, will it be because of one of those chemicals? Which chemical is the biggest problem? Or is it a combination of chemicals? The point of the data collection was likely to demonstrate that the next generation may be in danger because of their absorption of too many chemicals from the environment. Like much epidemiological data, it proves nothing specifically, but it does raise general concerns. Could these chemicals be causing higher cancer, autism, and/or allergy rates in this generation of children?

"We should try to reduce pesticide intake as much as possible," Dr. Firestone allows, "but it is complicated."

Aren't there standards and rules for pesticide use and residue? Of course there are, but the level of monitoring for compliance is suspect. A lawyer specializing in FDA regulations compliance whom I met at a meeting confided that because of budget restrictions, monitoring depends on the "squeal" program. In other words, your competitors squeal on you to the FDA if you are not behaving, acting like a large unpaid policing unit. The budget for monitoring compliance is "minuscule," Dr. Firestone confirms. "For example," he continues, "what fruit or vegetable do children eat the most?"

That is easy: apples, if you are counting applesauce and juice. He concurs, and I am still in the running for food *Jeopardy!*, but I sense a trick question coming up.

"Where do most apples in this country come from?" he continues.

"Washington State?" I reply tentatively.

"China," he sighs. "The land of things that never get tested."

In fact, according to a CNN report, 50 percent of the apple juice imported to the United States comes from China. The U.S. Apple Association claims that 47 percent of all the apples on the planet come from China.

The bottom line? It just seems to make logical sense to avoid as many toxins as you reasonably can, even though it may not yet be possible to link symptoms directly to pesticides.

DALE: THE PLOT THICKENS

Dale, an adorable three-year-old, came to me because her parents did not know what to do about her hives. They insisted Dale had been born with spots. For all of her short life, she had suffered from this rashlike skin condition that no one—not her pediatrician, not the dermatologist, not an infectious disease specialist, not an allergist—could get to the bottom of. She had tested negative to all allergies. And the hives were extensive. There was not a square inch of her skin that was hive-less. When I saw her, she was so red and bumpy that I had to force myself not to stare in fascination. Luckily, she seemed blissfully unaware of her unusual appearance and was a happy, social child. As toddlers, her preschool friends had not started asking her why she looked different, but her parents were painfully aware that those days were not long off.

When I took Dale's history, I learned that she was both nursed and given formula since birth. Because the hives had erupted at such a young age, I wondered if the cause was linked to something she had ingested in formula or breast milk. Her parents had been diligent about avoiding any other possible contaminants, such as ointments, soap, shampoo—anything at all that could have triggered a skin reaction. In addition, they had taken her off dairy products and eggs, and had never introduced gluten. They were trying to avoid the most common allergic foods since she clearly had problems and the tests had not illuminated a cause.

"How do you handle the itching?" I wanted to know.

"Her doctor prescribed antihistamine medication that we're supposed to give her twenty-four/seven," her father, Phil, answered. "We were not comfortable with that amount of medicine, so we only use it if she is really feeling bad. Since we took out dairy and eggs, she doesn't itch as much."

The clues looked like this:

- hives (red, itchy bumps) all over her body and face
- irritants had already been removed, including those in skin products and foods
- some use of antihistamines

I was stymied.

With Chuck, the chemicals used to treat the strawberries were the problem, not the food. Then I reviewed the most recent literature on pest control and saw that since the late 1990s, genetic engineering (GE) technology can tie the pesticide effect or other desirable growing traits into the DNA of the plant. GE is now commonly used to remove pieces of DNA from bacteria or viruses and insert them into plants. For example, 80 percent of corn now contains its own internal insecticide genetically engineered into its DNA. This corn is referred to as Bt corn, and all foods using this kind of technology are called genetically modified organisms (GMO). I asked myself, What if Dale's reaction could be tied to these newer internalized chemical alterations?

Even a fifth grader can tell you that a cow and an ear of corn cannot produce offspring, but we have walked around this little prohibition by taking pieces of genetic material from one part of the animal kingdom (bacteria and viruses) and artificially inserting it into the plant kingdom. The result is plants that, over the short run at least, resist bugs better (maybe because they are part bug). Dr. Frankenstein would have been proud, whereas Charles Darwin is probably turning over in his grave. We have scientifically achieved something heretofore impossible in nature: We have made animal plants. Hence the confusing term *genetically modified organism* referring to a plant.

Since the introduction of GMOs into the food supply in the 1990s, allergic reactions have been skyrocketing. According to Robyn O'Brien, author of *The Unhealthy Truth*, since genetically altered soy was introduced on a widespread scale in 1996, soy allergies have increased dramatically. Levels of major soy allergens are 27 percent higher in genetically modified soy, she contends. Likewise peanut allergies have risen 20 percent each year starting in 1997, again, the year after GMO soy started being widely consumed. Peanuts are in the same plant family as soy. Reactions to one food in a plant family can increase reactivity to other members of the same family. This is why people who are allergic to almonds often have trouble with other nuts. People do not think of soy and peanuts as being in the same botanical family, but they are both legumes grown in the ground. Therefore, anything that dramatically raises reactions to soy could increase problems with peanuts.

In 1999, the prestigious medical journal *The Lancet* reported that there has been a presumption that GE foods entail no greater risks of unexpected effects than conventional ones even though there are "good reasons to believe that specific risks may exist." The writers concluded that "governments should never have allowed these products into the food chain without insisting on rigorous testing for effects on health." But because of the unproven presumption of safety, they have.

When I first started my practice almost thirty years ago, corn allergies were unheard of. We never even put corn on the list of possible suspects.

BEYOND ORGANIC FOR THE ENVIRONMENTALLY CONSCIENTIOUS

It's great to buy organic, but there are other issues to consider as well—humanitarian treatment of both farm workers and animals and food's carbon footprint. Some farmers are taking steps to go "beyond organic." An organic tomato can be grown four thousand miles away by workers not being paid a living wage, for example. The more conscientious producers and consumers may want to consider the environmental impact of growing food out of season and trekking it halfway around the world, as well as the working conditions of the farm laborers.

The other concern is the living conditions of farm animals. Certified organically raised animals must have some outdoor access, although the amount is not defined. They must also be provided with bedding materials. The standards for the care of conventionally raised animals address food safety rather than animal comfort. Safe meat is important, but an enlightened culture also considers the welfare of its animals.

Today, corn and soy reactions are common. Most infant formulas contain both corn and soy. Because 80 percent of corn and 93 percent of soy is genetically modified, I hypothesized that Dale had had early exposure to GMOs and that they may have confused and disrupted her immune system. This was the basis of my theory.

"This might sound a little out there," I started telling her parents, "but I think we should take Dale off all corn and soy products and anything else that might contain a genetically modified substance."

Dale's parents listened intensely, their eyes getting wider and jaws dropping slowly. "Uh-oh," I thought. "They are going into shock and think this is crazy." I blindly babbled on, explaining how we would probably never prove the theory but it might help Dale get better. When I finally finished, they both stared at me for a few tense seconds and then smiled.

"It makes so much sense," the mother said. "Nobody has had any explanation to offer or any possible plan to follow except long-term medicine."

And just like that, they decided on an elimination trial, removing all foods that contained corn and soy from Dale's diet. The fact that she was an only child made it easier to make the dietary changes, because there were no other children's preferences to consider. Phil cleared his throat and confided that they would love to have another child but did not want to try unless Dale could be helped.

Taking out GMO food meant removing most processed food that did not contain organic ingredients. Cornstarch, corn syrup, soy oil, soy proteins, and other soy/corn derivatives are in all premade food. You almost have to assume a corn or soy derivative is there and that it is genetically modified unless otherwise specified. GMO food does not have to be labeled in this country, but certified organic food may not contain GMO ingredients. Dale's diet sounds like a throwback to *Little House on the Prairie*. It contains meat, fruits, vegetables, seeds, grains, and homemade baked goods. The ingredients are certified organic whenever possible.

Dale slowly started to improve over several months. Her itching went away completely and the hives faded some, but as of this writing, she is not completely cured. She still has too many bumps, but they do not itch. Her parents rarely need to give her medicine anymore, and Dale is thriving and developing normally in every way. As much as we like things to be cut and dried, the situation is rarely simple when it comes to GMOs and environmental toxins. If it were, we would have better safety data and a cleaner food supply. Nonetheless, Dale's parents believe they are on the right track and see a light at the end of this long, nightmarish tunnel. We are considering some new blood tests that would measure exposure to volatile solvents, chlorinated pesticides, parabens, and other environmental toxins. I suggested that perhaps we should test her mother, because the parents still hold that Dale was born with spots. The long, twisted quest continues, through which Dale's parents remain thankful. Despite a few dots and spots, Dale is one of the healthiest children around.

NUTRITION DETECTIVE PRINCIPLE #15

Not having proof of direct harm does not mean a product is safe.

Although there is mounting research that points to the harmful effects of chemicals, environmental toxins, and genetically modified foods, it's still difficult to trace the direct effect of substances that are present in most, if not all, conventionally grown foods. I suggest that you think about irritants in a broader way. Until we have better safety data and the national will to commit the resources necessary to monitor the food supply and label it completely, it is up to you, the parent, to protect your children. Buy the cleanest, least-altered food you can afford. Be ready to commit more financial resources to your food budget. As a country, we are accustomed to plentiful, cheap food. But we should also insist on safe food produced in a way that protects the environment, even if it costs more money. Every dollar spent on organic food is one less dollar needed down the road to clean up the pesticide runoff killing fish in the Chesapeake Bay or at the doctor's office trying to figure out your child's hard-to-diagnose health issue.

ARTIFICIAL COLORINGS

The tales of Chuck and Dale illustrate potential reactions to pesticides and GMO, but a chapter on suspicious substances added to food would not be complete without a word about synthetic food colorings. Bright colors are often added to kiddie food to make the macaroni-and-cheese look cheesier or the juice drink look more appealing. Synthetic food colors are cheaper, easier to use, and more vibrant than natural hues, hence their popularity with food manufacturers. Nine dyes are approved in the United States for food use. They are Blue 1, Blue 2, Citrus Red 2, Green 3, Orange B, Red 3, Red 40, Yellow 5, and Yellow 6, in case you become a *Who Wants to Be a Millionaire?* contestant and this question comes up.

These substances are all capable of causing skin and allergic reactions in children, so they should be added to the list of possible irritants if your child is itching or develops a rash. This is well known enough that allergy medicine can be purchased without dye so that allergic people do not react to the medicine that is supposed to be helping their reaction.

The bigger controversy about dye involves whether or not it negatively affects behavior. The same debate that plagues sugar's potential effect on children's behavior hangs over the synthetic dye issue. Parents and doctors complain that some children's behavior gets worse when they eat food with dye, although the FDA and food industry dismiss these claims as unproven. In 2004, the results of fifteen studies concluded there was a modest worsening of behavior when children with ADHD consumed foods with synthetic dyes.

Since then, the British government has commissioned two studies to clarify the situation. The study results were convincing enough that the European Union passed a law requiring a warning notice on foods that contain one or more of six suspicious dyes. The warning reads, "May have an adverse effect on activity and attention on children." You may wish to heed that warning.

Does Your Child React to Pesticides or GMOs?

It can be difficult to tell whether a reaction is to the food itself or something sprayed on it, genetically tied into it, or added later. To figure it out, ask yourself these questions.

☐ Does your child get symptoms sometimes but not others when eating the same food? For example, did she have grapes last week with no ill effects, but this week she has a rash? Or, did she eat applesauce with no problem, but got an itchy throat eating an apple?

☐ Does your child have red cheeks or rashes that come and go in a way that makes it impossible to find a trigger food?

☐ Is your child highly sensitive in other ways? To sounds, lights, or temperature, for example? Children who are more sensory sensitive have more delicate nervous systems and may be more reactive to toxins.

☐ Does your child sometimes complain of an itchy throat or mouth?

☐ Does your child seem to be allergic to something but allergy testing comes up negative?

Answering yes to any of these questions may mean that your child is having a negative reaction to something besides the food itself, most likely to pesticide residues, artificial flavors or colors, or genetically modified food.

What to Do

The simplest thing is to choose organic food as often as possible.

According to regulations implemented in 2002 by the U.S. Department of Agriculture, organic food and beverage products need to be grown without the use of genetically engineered seeds, growth hormones, sewage sludge, or irradiation. The use of toxic pesticides and fertilizers is also prohibited, but some organically grown food may have pesticide residue owing to drift from surrounding areas.

Some simple tips:

1. Buy local. Talk to the purveyors at your local farmers' market. Although they may not all be certified organic, their growing practices and proximity may make their products a good choice nonetheless. One group of Amish farmers at our local market uses no pesticides at their farm, although they have not gotten organic certification,

citing "too much red tape." At least that is what I think they said. My Pennsylvania Dutch is not what it used to be.

2. **Watch your meat and dairy.** The most important foods to buy organic are meat and dairy products, especially cheese and butter. At the top of the food chain, animal products consistently contain the highest pesticide residues.

3. **Know the dirty dozen.** If you cannot afford to buy all of your food organic or if availability is low, it helps to know which fruits and vegetables are best and worst when it comes to pesticide residues. Concentrate on the items with the lowest amounts of pesticide residue when investing your organic dollars. According to the Environmental Working Group (EWG), there are four basic categories, ordered left to right from worst to best (see the table at right).

   The closer to the left a food item is on the chart, the harder you should try to buy only organic for that item. In particular, avoid nonorganic purchases from the two left columns, especially the farthest left. Some pesticides are taken up internally by the plants and find their way into the parts of the plant you eat; thus, the pesticides cannot be washed off. Other pesticides are designed to bind tightly to the surface of the fruit or vegetable so rain doesn't wash them off, which means you cannot easily wash them off, either. Even the foods listed in the far right column were not always found to be pesticide-free, but they were consistently low in pesticide residues and are your best bets for nonorganic food.

   An EWG simulation showed that people can lower their pesticide exposure 90 percent by avoiding the most contaminated fruits and vegetables. It may be tempting to think you can "beat the list" by extra washing and peeling, but the fruits and vegetables listed opposite were treated as they would be by a careful consumer. For instance, bananas were peeled and apples were washed before testing. Peeling does reduce exposure to surface-level pesticides for many of these foods, but you often lose valuable nutrients and roughage when you throw away the peel. And how are you going to peel spinach or a strawberry?

THE RED ZONE AVOID UNLESS ORGANIC	SO-SO LEVELS . . . SO USE CAUTION	BETTER . . . BUT NOT PERFECT	AHH . . . BEST OF THE BUNCH
• peaches	• spinach	• applesauce	• broccoli
• apples	• grapes	• raspberries	• orange juice
• sweet bell peppers	• lettuce	• plums	• blueberries
• celery	• potatoes	• grapefruit	• papaya
• nectarines	• green beans	• tangerine	• cabbage
• strawberries	• hot peppers	• apple juice	• bananas
• cherries	• cucumbers	• honeydew melon	• kiwi
• carrots	• mushrooms	• tomatoes	• canned tomatoes
• pears	• cantaloupe	• sweet potatoes	• sweet peas
• frozen winter squash	• oranges	• watermelon	• asparagus
	• fresh winter squash	• cauliflower	• mango
			• canned pears
			• pineapple
			• sweet corn
			• avocado
			• onions

It's also important to remember that the best-to-worst list applies not only to fresh fruits and vegetables, but often to the same items when they are canned or frozen, as well as to processed foods and restaurant meals.

4. Avoid GMOs. The four big GMOs are corn, soy, canola, and cotton-seed oil. Companies in the United States are not required to disclose the use of GMOs, so unless otherwise labeled, assume any prepared food containing any of these ingredients has a genetically engineered component. Foods certified organic, even as an ingredient on a bottle or box, by definition should be GMO-free. Some nonorganic foods will label their products "GMO-free," so keep any eye out for that.

For further information, check out the non-GMO shopping guide available at www.nongmoshoppingguide.com/SG/Home/index.cfm. There is also more information at www.centerforfoodsafety.org.

CHAPTER 16

The Child Who Couldn't Speak in Sentences

A S PARENTS, WE WATCH IN awe and anticipation as our babies reach their milestones: the first smile, the first step, the first sleep through the night. We are exceptionally interested in how and when they utter their first words. A *mama* or *gaga* can make us simply melt. Conversely, when our kids aren't hitting the speaking milestones, we can worry . . . and we should.

Adam was four and a half when I first started working with him and his family. He was an adorable, polite child who seemed eager to please, although he did not say much. "Say hello, Adam," his mother, Paola, prompted, and he complied immediately but without elaboration. He sat on the floor and started playing happily with an assortment of toys I keep in my office. I asked Adam if he would mind if his mother and I talked about him, and he said, "Okay" without looking up.

Paola confirmed that talking in his presence would not cause him undue stress. "I just wanted you to see him," she blurted. "You can see he is a wonderful child, but he does not talk much." She went on to fill in the details of his story.

WORDS WITHOUT SPEECH

Adam's early life was pretty uneventful. He was born on time after an easy pregnancy. He had some trouble latching on, so breast-feeding was difficult, but his mother persisted, using formula to supplement her breast milk. His easy disposition made him a family favorite, and he thrived developmentally and physically until he was between the ages of two and a half and three.

At some point, Paola started suspecting that not everything was as it should be. Adam pointed to what he wanted. He also was able to echo any word back to the speaker, much to the delight of his parents. But his language was not evolving toward complexity. By the time Adam was three, Paola was convinced that saying "juice" or "want juice" instead of "May I have some juice, please?" was not enough. His language skills were not on par with those of his peers.

She had him evaluated through a county screening program. Early intervention programs are federally mandated but locally administered throughout the country. The testing identified a functional language delay, but it was not serious enough for Adam to qualify for free services. "He understands everything," the tester assured Paola. "He will be fine."

Paola was not convinced. She prodded Adam to say complete sentences. "Say, 'May I have juice, please?' " she would insist before handing over the requested item. He would repeat whatever she said, but the next time, the request went back to the stripped-down version. Frustrated, Paola pursued private speech therapy. After months of therapy, Adam started using two- and three-word phrases more frequently, but the progress was very slow. Now at four and a half, Adam struggled to string a sentence together and was not conversational. If asked a "what" or "why" question, he would just say, "No, thank you."

A second problem was also emerging: behavior. As the gap between Adam's communication ability and that of his peers widened, anxiety and frustration started to drive antisocial behavior. Adam badly wanted to play with other children, but the words would not come out, so he tried yelling and pushing to get his point across. His parents knew Adam's acting out was directly related to his poor communication skills and wanted to help him, but behavior modification was not working. Medication was recommended to help improve his frustration tolerance, but Adam was only four years old and Paola wanted to explore a do-no-harm approach first.

WHEN SPEECH IS DELAYED

The technical term for Adam's problem is *speech dyspraxia*. Break down *dyspraxia* and you get *dys* and *praxia*. The prefix *dys* means "off" or "not." A *dys*functional family is an off or not functional family. *Praxia* or *praxis* means "movement." Put them together and you get what the Dyspraxia Foundation defines as "the impairment or immaturity of the organization of movement." Usually developmental dyspraxia is tied to the motor planning of how a child moves around. Does he lack the coordination to ride a bike or is he clumsy on the playground? If so, perhaps he has a developmental coordination disorder or motor dyspraxia.

Few of us consider how important good motor planning is in our everyday activities. It occurs to you that you need a book from across the room and you go get it. Plans are not made and little conscious thought is involved. But many complex neurological and motor operations are needed to perform such a simple task easily. One foot has to be put in front of the other. Your arm movements must be controlled. Balance needs to be maintained. In addition, obstacles ("Watch out for that ottoman!") have to be circumvented. The list goes on and on. Even a basic skill like walking some distance and picking up an object requires good motor planning, and when the skill is mastered, nobody has to think about it.

Now imagine that your legs do not respond reliably when you need them and you are not sure exactly how to get to the book without tripping. Then you realize your arms are not balancing you properly and you have to think about what to do with them. All of a sudden, picking up a book across the room is a whole lot of trouble, which is what it is like when a person has movement motor planning and coordination problems (dyspraxia).

The other type of dyspraxia involves speech and the motor planning of talking. At the most basic level of speech motor planning, a child knows a word and pulls it out at the appropriate time. Instead of getting a book across the room, this time he is retrieving a word in his brain. This basic motor planning of speech develops without issues in most children, just as most kids can easily run across the playground and pick up an object. "What's this?" the parent asks, and the child says "A cow" or "A V-8–powered fuel-injected classic Corvette with a dual exhaust system" if he is a boy. Kids with speech dyspraxia have a much more difficult time with word retrieval and the other processes involved with speech. In extreme cases, which are called apraxia, there is little or no unprompted speech. The child may understand the words but cannot find, retrieve, and say them.

As language evolves in complexity, the process requires more motor planning and additional parts of the brain need to be coordinated. Answering "What's this?" requires a quick word retrieval. "What did you do at school today?" requires a more complex answer. It involves finding the words, prioritizing thoughts, deciding what is relevant to report, and organizing a response. Is the answer to that question "I like yellow"? No. Prioritizing for relevance, which happens in a different part of the brain than basic language, discounts this response. How about "Nothing" or "I don't know"? If a teenager is muttering them, all is completely normal, but if a five-year-old uses these monosyllabic responses exclusively, they are a request for help in organizing (motor planning) an answer. If the parent follows with, "Did you have music or art today?" often the child can answer with more details.

Adam said, "No, thank you" when asked a complex question because he was conscious enough to know it required an answer, but could not generate an appropriate response, so he used a comfortable and acceptable script. He had individual words, but lacked the motor planning to put them together in a conversation. Interestingly, the motor coordination center is right next to the speech center in the brain, and they are intricately connected. We walk before we talk because development of the movement center drives development of the speech. Movement drives speech, which is why children often talk more when they are swinging in a swing or jumping up and down. Consequently, motor coordination and speech dyspraxia often occur together in children.

When children are speech delayed, interventional therapy should be the first line of attack. Early screening and intervention programs are available across the country and widely recognized as critical for later academic success. Yet, unless the child is living in poverty and not eating, not a word is said about the biochemical environment that sets up learning. Without the right nutrients, some children will not have the proper

A CLOSER LOOK AT DYSPRAXIA

D r. Marilyn Agin is a neurodevelopmental pediatrician, the former medical director of the New York City Early Intervention program, and the coauthor of *The Late Talker*. Before developing an expertise in dyspraxia, she was a speech-language pathologist. When asked, "What do you believe parents need to know about dyspraxia?" she offered the following:

When parents bring their child for an evaluation, usually the primary concern is delayed speech and language development. They need to know that the development of the motor system is critical in the development of the whole child. Everything else builds on that foundation. It is not uncommon for a child with low muscle tone to also have weak postural stability. (Postural stability is the ability to maintain an upright posture and balance, and is the "core" or basis of other motor skills.) Without a stable "core," there

will be a general weakness in oral motor skills, including trouble with chewing, swallowing, and tongue movement, as well as other gross- and fine-motor delays that affect overall movement and speech output. In my experience, if you look carefully, most children with apraxia of speech have an associated motor dyspraxia, also known as "clumsy child syndrome."

To overcome dyspraxia, a task needs to be broken down into small units. Eventually, after many repetitions, it becomes learned and automatic. It's like learning to play tennis. Yes, there are the natural athletes who can watch someone play and easily learn to volley, but most of us need the skill broken down into discrete steps that need to be executed over and over again. With apraxia and dyspraxia of speech, children are hearing the language, but they don't know how to get started, get the words from their brain to their mouths, and then organize the sequence of movements to form words and phrases. If we

brain chemistry to allow them to acquire the skills no matter how many speech therapy sessions they have.

IS MY CHILD JUST CLUMSY OR DYSPRAXIC?

Dyspraxia is one symptom of many for a number of medical conditions, including cerebral palsy, muscular dystrophy, and mitochondrial disorders. (Mitochondrial disorders are a group of

identify these children early and teach using lots of repetition, most can become verbal communicators.

The incidence appears to be increasing in a parallel fashion to autism. In some children, we can identify a genetic component that is most probably triggered by exposure to environmental toxins or allergens. We are learning as we go, but given the fact that we come into contact with so many environment hazards such as pesticides, we are likely triggering some rather unhelpful recessive genes.

Developmental issues often get short shrift in pediatric practice because of the sheer number of issues the general pediatrician has to deal with in a fifteen-minute well-child visit. Inadequate training of practitioners and lack of insurance reimbursement for developmental screening contribute to the problem of missed opportunities in identifying children with developmental delays by the primary care provider. Early identification of apraxia and dyspraxia

is key to paving the way for better long-term educational and social outcomes for our children.

Again, you would be surprised how often parents are told to "just wait six months and she will be fine" when they raise a concern about a child with a speech delay. The difference between delays that will likely sort themselves out on their own and dyspraxia is not always obvious. More than that, it is often missed by very busy pediatricians. For more in-depth information on dyspraxia, read Dr. Agin's book *The Late Talker.*

You would think picking up apraxia in a child, which basically means they are not saying any words, would be an obvious "duh" to any pediatrician, but it is not. For unclear reasons, there is a tendency to make excuses for delays: "Check in again in six months and let's see." Or, "Boys [or twins or third children] are often late talkers." The ability to tell the difference between children who will likely sort themselves out without help and those with dyspraxia/ apraxia takes training and skill.

conditions that interfere with the way the body turns food into energy that cells can use.) Although dyspraxia is a specific learning disability, it is not associated with low intelligence or predictive of overall learning potential by itself. Dyspraxia USA (www.dyspraxiausa.com), an advocacy group committed to raising awareness and helping those living with the condition, estimates that the number of children with dyspraxia falls somewhere between 6 and 20 percent. Such a large incidence range can be blamed on the broad areas dyspraxia encompasses coupled with imprecise diagnosing techniques. Six to 20 percent includes speech, fine-motor, and whole-body movement disorders. For example, a child having trouble writing and holding a pencil (a fine-motor problem) but with no other issues would be included in that number.

For gross, or whole-body movement dyspraxia, symptoms include poor balance, awkward or incorrect sequencing of movements, poor spatial awareness (bumping into objects and people), trouble keeping left and right straight, an inability to cross the body's midline, difficulties remembering what to do next motorwise, and the ever famous inability to combine two motor activities (such as walk and chew gum).

We take for granted many of these basic processes, so often that people do not understand what some of them mean. Let me explain. Incorrect movement sequencing is exactly what it sounds like: making mistakes when deciding the order of movements. A child trying to catch a ball may put her foot out instead of putting her arms up, and as a result, the ball hits her in the chest. Crossing midline is literally the ability to move your arm farther than halfway across the front of the body. Imagine the restrictive and odd movements you would have if you could move each arm only to the middle of your body. Without this skill, for example, children will write to the middle of a page and then move down to the next line or switch the pencil to the other hand to continue. Finally, having trouble with remembering what to do next (i.e., your motor skills) means having to think through basic maneuvers every time you do them. How do I open a peanut butter jar, again?

Because dyspraxia often travels with other conditions such as speech delay, memory problems, sensory processing disorder, dyslexia, and ADHD, teasing it out as a separate condition can be messy and has also caused fruitless debates about what to call the symptom. A precise dyspraxia diagnosis from a specialist is not necessary. For example, clumsiness becomes dyspraxia when a parent, teacher, or developmental specialist notices it is part of a group of movement symptoms interfering with normal learning and development. Speech delays become dyspraxia to me when the language is in the brain and is not being expressed smoothly, easily, or in the right order.

Once, I watched a six-year-old lean over to pick up a toy and fall into a wall. We all execute an embarrassing motor blunder now and again, but what was different about this incident was the extreme level of concentration the child needed to attempt this simple movement and the awkward sequence of movements she used. An observer could predict the coming disaster based on the bad decisions she was making about where to put her arms and legs. I was not surprised to learn from her mother that she injured herself on a regular basis. That is dyspraxia.

WHAT IS THE RIGHT CHEMISTRY FOR LEARNING?

Nobody knows exactly how people learn, but we do know that when you learn something, the chemistry of the neurons (brain cells) used for the new skill changes in response to their frequent activation. For example, say the talent scout calls from *Dancing with the Stars*. You are thrilled but have not danced since you were in your high school production of *The Pajama Game*. When the choreographer instructs you to shimmy, the neurons in your motor cortex associated with trunk movement fire in a way that they haven't done since 1994. Now you are telling them to bend this and shake that, and the neuron firing sequence associated with these movements is activated. The result feels awkward and looks worse.

So you practice and fire that neuron sequence over and over, many hours a day, for many weeks running. At a certain point of repetition, the neurons start to change. This is a busy, important pathway, the brain decides. Let's build a better connecting circuit. Neurons that never passed information to each other before start to communicate. More receptor sites appear and calcium concentrations shift to make firing easier. Remember how the brain turns chemical energy into electrical impulses?

Calcium is called an electrolyte because it can be used to generate electricity, and its concentration and movement are critical for sending signals in the brain.

As language grows, more neural connections are needed to accomplish more sophisticated operations.

In a busy part of the brain, one neuron can have 100,000 connections, but neurons do not start with this many. Every time you learn a new skill or have a new experience, you increase the number of connections that some of your neurons have to others. On the outside, you start to look like less of a klutz, because on the inside, the brain has been building new and better pathways. The left foot follows the right foot without thinking about each step. Your brain chemistry has shifted, and you have learned to dance like a pro.

Now substitute learning to talk for learning to dance. A similar sequence of chemical events happens, albeit in different parts of the brain. Another difference is that there are expected stages of language development. In *Dancing with the Stars*, who knows if Marie Osmond can learn the samba or what the result will look like. With language, however, there is a distinct predictable sequence of mastery. First there is babbling and sound imitation. This leads to word approximations and real words. Then the child starts putting words together using verbs and adding pronouns. Up to this point the language is mostly about demands ("Want juice" or "Don't want carrot") or observations ("See airplane"). Most children quickly figure out basic sentence structure next ("I want to go outside now"). Then they move to reciprocal language or the ability to respond to other people's input. Finally, language acquires abstract characteristics so the child can answer why questions, use imagination, and subtly manipulate it for her own purposes. ("I don't need a nap because I took one yesterday").

The brain becomes more complex as language grows. More connections are needed to accomplish more sophisticated operations. When there is a developmental delay or learning disability, the child has an experience but it does not get tied into the neurons and learned. He can be exposed to the same concept or information over and over but not master it.

The right chemistry supports learning so that the neurons, when stimulated by new experiences, can work together across their many and varied networks in an appropriate manner. Brain chemistry is influenced by experiences, genetics, and environmental elements, and the environmental factor we can best control and manipulate is the diet.

A gigantic number of nutritional factors influence the chemistry of learning, but I am going to concentrate on three, because after years of experimentation, I have found that they make the most dramatic improvements the most efficiently. They are all in the fat family. Why fats? The brain is mostly fat, so the fats you take in become the building blocks of the brain. Fats are structural nutrients. If you took a brain to a chemist and asked her to tell you what it was made of, she would tell you most of it (60–70 percent) is fat.

When rats are fed a diet high in the kind of fats found in a typical fast-food meal of a burger or nuggets and fries, they cannot learn how to run through mazes. At the end of these studies, the researchers chop off the heads of the animals and study the brains, which have early signs of the same type of neuron tangles found in Alzheimer's disease. Yes, it is gruesome, but it is also the reason we know more about rat diets than our own. Why is this information relevant? Because kids are eating those same kinds of fats every day, but we cannot peer into their brains and see how incorporating those fats into the brain is affecting learning. Plus, for humans, learning is much more complex, so we cannot plop kids in a maze and use their performance as a total measure of learning. What we do know for sure is that the right fats are critical for learning.

Beyond the essential fats and fish oils discussed previously, I have worked with some other types of fats that are important to brain function and learning and designed a specific biochemical booster plan geared toward motor planning. I have taught therapists, doctors, and parents all over the country how to use my strategy, which I have boldly named "The Best Dyspraxia Program Ever." As a title, "The Best Dyspraxia Program Ever" is over the top, but the name is intentionally outlandish to get people's attention, because motor planning is important for so many types of learning issues.

THE BEST DYSPRAXIA PROGRAM EVER

I have been talking so much about dyspraxia that you have probably forgotten all about Adam. Unlike many of the children you have met throughout this book, Adam was a good eater. My heart soared as I looked at the diet diary Paola provided. He ate vegetables and fruit every day along with a few servings of dairy products. He also ate whole grains, the occasional bean dish, and lean meat.

There was not much mystery to the polite child sitting in my office. He was a perfect candidate for my program. His diet was strong, so I could concentrate on what might be missing. How could something be missing when the diet is strong? Bio-individuality. For reasons not entirely clear, some children need much more than the average amount of nutrients for learning. Or perhaps more accurately, they seem to respond well to the addition of large amounts of certain nutrients. The hope was that the right biochemical support for language learning would help him improve his limited speech skills and get him back on track.

Here are the three parts of the program:

1. The omega-3 fatty acids eicosapentaenoic acid (EPA) and docosahexaenoic acid (DHA) or fish oil

2. Vitamin E complex

3. Phosphatidylcholine (PC)

Fish Oil. I've touted the benefits of fish oil in other chapters (see pages 181–182 and 213–215), but they bear repeating: Fish oil can help with ADHD and mood, and now we add dyspraxia. Many studies have found specific benefits of omega-3 fatty acids for motor planning. Most products are a combination of EPA and DHA (see "How to Read Fish Oil Labels" on page 144). After age three, a therapeutic amount of a combination of EPA and DHA starts at about 1,000 milligrams. There is no risk of toxicity with fish oil. If a child consumes more than she can digest, the oils will cause loose stools.

Vitamin E is a fat-soluble antioxidant, so it belongs in the fat family. Antioxidants donate electrons to unstable molecules to make them happy, or more "stable," in chemical lingo. Molecules can become unstable as a result of injury, toxin exposure, and malnutrition, as well as for other reasons. Vitamin E is designed to operate in parts of the body that are fat-based, such as the brain. There are both water- and fat-based substances in the body, so you need antioxidants for both mediums. Vitamin C is the most famous example of a water-based antioxidant.

Claudia Morris, a California pediatrician, discovered that many children with dyspraxia show symptoms of vitamin E deficiency. The symptoms of vitamin E deficiency are slow language development, abnormal proprioception, a high pain threshold, low muscle tone, and poor motor coordination and planning. Proprioception is your sense of your body in space. Proprioceptor ability is what the police are testing when they pull over suspected drunk drivers; they want to see if the driver is able to maintain balance and walk a straight line. Normal proprioception would not require looking at the line or your feet to walk straight.

Vitamin E, which is found in wheat germ oil, almonds, and oils such as safflower, corn, and soy, is notoriously low in the diets of American children, who in general don't get the minimum recommended levels. Few people eat wheat germ oil (the best source), but they might ingest some vitamin E if they are eating whole wheat or other whole grains, which retain some of the germ.

As a result of Dr. Morris's observations, many professionals have started recommending vitamin E, in addition to fish oil, for dyspraxic children.

Vitamin E is completely nontoxic, but in high doses can cause blood thinning. Starting at age three, 800 IUs is usually enough to create a therapeutic effect, but is not high enough to cause most children to bruise easily. Doctors using more aggressive dosing will run a one-time blood test to be sure the high levels of vitamin E are not affecting clotting time. Vitamin E has eight components, including four tocotrienols and four tocopherols. Look for a complete vitamin E complex with alpha, beta, delta, and gamma tocopherols, plus tocotrienols. Vitamin E complex at these dosing levels is found only in capsules, so if your child is not yet swallowing pills, be prepared to puncture a few and squeeze them out. A parent can swallow the shell of the capsule and reap the benefits of taking a small amount of vitamin E.

Phosphatidylcholine (PC). *Phosphatidylcholine* is a mouthful—you can impress your less biochemically oriented friends if you can pronounce it correctly and use it in a sentence. It is part of a family of compounds called phospholipids that are the building blocks of all cell membranes. The job of the phospholipids is to provide a barrier between the outside and the inside of the cell, so the extracellular stuff does not mix inappropriately with the intracellular materials. The phospholipids line up along the outside wall of the cell like little support posts holding the cells together.

Because one end of the phospholipid molecule likes water and the other likes fat, they literally help the body—which is made up of these two opposing substances—stick together. Without enough PC, the cells, particularly in the brain, fall apart and die. Whether anyone's level of PC has actually been so low that their brain started breaking down, I do not know, but I suspect it is exceedingly rare. There is a lot of territory between dire deficiency and optimal functioning. From the results I have witnessed when supplemental PC is given, I presume children's learning is affected from not having enough.

How does PC affect motor planning and language? PC is not only an important structural component of the brain but also the building block of acetylcholine, a neurotransmitter that regulates memory, motor planning, and executive functions such as sorting and prioritizing. Found in beef and chicken livers (best sources), eggs, lean ground beef, and peanut butter, choline (as part

NEURON FACTOIDS FOR NERDS

Neurons come in different shapes and sizes and are classified by their shape, location, and function. Some interesting facts about neurons:

- The average number of neurons in a person is 100 billion.
- Fetuses grow neurons at a rate of 250,000 per minute.
- The speed of a signal transmitted along a neuron is 1.2 to 250 miles per hour.

of PC) is critical for brain development. In 1998 the National Academy of Science recognized choline as an essential nutrient and established a daily requirement. Not until 2004 did the U.S. Department of Agriculture (USDA) publish a database for food sources of choline. The deficiency symptom for choline is a reduced capacity to learn. Because it's an essential nutrient, choline needs to be ingested and then it can be used to make other important molecules. Other nutrients, such as folic acid, are needed so the basic nutrient choline can be used to build complex substances such as acetylcholine and PC.

Although it's possible to eat choline so your body can make PC, there's always the possibility of something going wrong when building molecules in the body, so my preference is to provide, when possible, the substance already made. Although it tastes disgusting, PC is available as a dietary supplement as a liquid or in large gel capsules. Usually it is derived from soy oil. If your child has a soy allergy, use PC with caution. Even though there is little soy protein (the allergic part) in PC products, highly reactive kids may still have issues. I recommend a highly concentrated liquid product containing 3,000 milligrams of PC for children age three and up. Only a few companies are making such a product, and it is expensive.

This flood-the-brain-with-the-critical-nutrient-and-hope-it-will-know-how-to-use-it technique has been shockingly successful, as you will see. The trickiest part is finding something thick and sweet to cover PC's goat-vomit taste. Despite its famously awful flavor, some children come to crave it and take it straight. The results have been so consistently good that finding a way to get the PC in is usually worth the trouble. If the child tolerates dairy products, yogurt works best. Straight honey or yogurt substitutes, such as coconut yogurt, may suffice, as well as drizzling the PC on a pancake and then putting a little syrup on top. In desperate cases, parents have melted chocolate, folded it in, and then cooled little chocolate pieces laced with PC on wax paper. Notice all the suggestions are thick and sweet.

> The results have been so consistently good that finding a way to get the PC in is usually worth the trouble.

For specific dosing information for any of the above supplements or before starting any supplement regimen, talk to your child's pediatrician or a qualified health care professional. If you start your child on supplements and she develops symptoms, stop them and see a physician.

Adam is one of many children who have blossomed on the three-fat dyspraxia support program. The fats do not all taste good and can be tricky to get in, but within months he was a completely different child. Because Adam could tolerate dairy products, Paola just folded all the fats into yogurt, which Adam gobbled up. She added one (the fish oil) the first week, then the vitamin E, and finally during week three, the PC oil.

Beatrice, another mother whose child was on the Best Dyspraxia Program Ever, told me her son took the PC and fish oils straight. She was convinced her son knew the supplements were helping and consequently was happy to take them off the spoon. Remember those commercials where they advise, "Do not try this at home"? Well, some mothers have tried this at home, and shockingly, it sometimes works. I would not advise it.

After two months on the program, Paola reported back. She was ecstatic when she related a story of how Adam explained to her how one of his toys worked. He went from a few clipped sentences to, "You know, Mom, you are supposed to put the . . ." She said her jaw was on the floor, while he acted as though he had always been talking at this level. Whether or not your child has a specific diagnosis of dyspraxia, if you think there is language trapped inside him just needing to break out, talk to your health care professional about incorporating the components of the Best Dyspraxia Program Ever.

WHEN FISH OIL DOESN'T WORK

Fish oil can work wonders, but unfortunately, not all learning issues or cases of dyspraxia can be solved by simply adding it or another omega-3 fatty acid supplement to the diet. Abadi, a three-year-old boy from a traditional Indian vegetarian family, was a case in point. He came to see me because of a developmental speech delay. Abadi had already been evaluated through a county early intervention program and was found to be significantly behind his peers.

After reading about the miraculous properties of omega-3 fats and realizing he was not getting these oils because of their vegetarian diet, his parents started giving him a fish oil supplement. Although they were vegetarians, they were willing to try anything to help Abadi. There was a clear result, but it was not the one they were expecting. Abadi immediately became cranky and out of control. His entire personality changed for the worse. They stopped the supplement immediately and decided to see a professional.

Although Abadi was not talking, he was interactive. As usual, I did my food diary inventory (see page 89) and found that Abadi was a pretty good eater. The traditional Indian diet is generally a healthy one. Abadi was eating dahl (lentils), vegetables, rice, fruit, and yogurt.

Then I looked at the big clue: an extreme reaction to a generally benign substance. Why would a child react so badly to a supplement that

273

NUTRITION DETECTIVE PRINCIPLE #16

Function follows structure.

This basic architecture principle is as true for the body as it is for a building. Providing the best building materials means the child can create the soundest structure for optimal functioning. One of the most important functions of the brain is learning, which is by and large a chemical process. Parents spend thousands of dollars for top-notch speech therapists and tutors but do not invest the same energy in the wires they are trying to plug in. Lauren Zimet, an Atlanta-based speech therapist, regularly recommends nutritional support for children in her practice. "In addition to speech therapy, nutritional support is key," she asserts. "I am continually amazed and inspired by the benefits of speech therapy in conjunction with nutritional support for the treatment of many speech and language disorders, not only dyspraxia." A child's capacity to learn has a lot to do with what is available biochemically. A typical child can develop normally with a balanced diet. A child with delays will need a good diet plus extra materials to close the developmental gap.

is usually well tolerated? As medical professionals, the first choice of response is a positive reaction where the symptoms improve. The second choice, believe it or not, is a negative response, because any response is better than none. Assuming the reaction is not serious (and they usually are not with nutritional supplements), any response means the vital nutrient you are testing is having a biological effect, and an experienced professional can use that information to move forward. However, you cannot steer a parked car. When a child walks into a practitioner's office and is taking a slew of targeted nutritional supplements and there has been no change in his condition (neither positive nor negative), chances are the solution to the problem is not in the realm of nutrition.

Decades of watching children means I have seen just about everything. I have seen Abadi's particular reaction a handful of times and worked out a theory about the underlying cause. My theory is the child is unable to digest and absorb fat properly, and the by-products of this poor digestion make the child feel bad and therefore act out. There are two reasons for poor digestion and absorption of fat in these cases: The child lacks the proper fat digestive enzymes, or the child needs more of an obscure nutrient called taurine.

Adding extra fat as a supplement is like a fat-digestion stress test. Abadi failed the test, but his stools were not yellow, extra-stinky, or loose, so I decided the problem was not insufficient digestive enzymes. I added a supplement taurine to improve fat uptake by the liver. The results? Abadi starting talking within a week! After nine months of proper supplements along with speech therapy, he was back in a regular preschool.

Why was this result so remarkable? It is likely that Abadi was not using the fat in his diet for brain development. The brain is mostly fat, so what you do with fat dramatically affects the brain. When his parents stressed him by adding more fat, the weakness in the system became apparent, and we were able to address it by adding 500 milligrams of taurine to his diet in the form of a supplement.

Taurine is not an essential nutrient, because it can be made from the proteins methionine and cysteine. It is a major component of bile, which is needed to process fat, but is also found in the white blood cells, nervous system, and muscles (including the heart). If you want to eat taurine, meat and fish are the major sources, and consequently, vegans tend to be low in taurine. Abadi was a vegetarian, and this may have contributed to his needing more than he got from his otherwise excellent diet. Although we know adults manufacture taurine, there is some debate about whether infants can, which is why it is added to infant formula.

How did I know to use taurine and not enzymes or indeed that fat utilization was the problem at all? This is where loads of observation and clinical experience come in handy. At first, I had never heard about what to do in a situation of a child not being able to digest fish oil, but once I ran into it a few times, I looked for similar characteristics and experimented with a few theories. You would be surprised at what kinds of creative solutions you can devise when you observe and are open to possibilities. Abadi's parents contributed by following through and getting help when their experiment did not go well. And we caught Abadi just in time: If he had come in at, say, six years old, we probably would not have been as successful at correcting his speech delay.

Is Your Child's Speech Delayed?

The first question to ask yourself is whether or not your child is speech delayed. The following milestone measures can help you decide if your child is developmentally on track for speech, or if there is a problem that nutritional supplements could help.

Cause for concern at twelve months:

☐ Easily upset by sounds that do not upset others

☐ May look at a desired object but does not clearly indicate that she wants it

☐ Not consistently babbling. Early babbling involves repeating sounds like "bababa," "mamama."

☐ Does not respond to words or gestures (for example, ignores hand motion to "come here")

☐ Does not understand language unless it is in context (for example, needs to see the cup when asked "want juice?")

Cause for concern at eighteen months:

☐ Understands fewer than fifty words

☐ Speaks fewer than ten words

☐ Does not attempt to imitate or spontaneously produce single words to convey meaning

☐ Has not increased vocabulary between twelve and eighteen months of age

Cause for concern at twenty-four months:

☐ Relies on gestures without verbalization

☐ Does not use two-word combinations

☐ Largely unintelligible speech

☐ Regression in language development, stops talking or begins echoing phrases, often inappropriate

☐ Speaks fewer than fifty words

Cause for concern at thirty-six months:

☐ Words limited to single syllables with no final consonants

☐ Few or no multiword utterances

☐ Does not demand a response from listeners

☐ Asks no questions

☐ Hard to understand

☐ Frequent tantrums when not understood

☐ Echoes or parrots speech rather than choosing what to say

Adapted with permission from *The Late Talker: What to Do If Your Child Isn't Talking Yet*, by Marilyn C. Agin, MD., Lisa Geng, and Malcolm Nicholl.

What to Do

1. The first step if you suspect speech delay based on these criteria is to have your child evaluated by a pediatric speech pathologist so the proper corrective therapy can be started ASAP. All states have free developmental screening programs, because early intervention can prevent learning issues later. If your state provides free services only for severe delays and you believe your child needs more help, as Adam's mother did, consider private therapy. Some medical insurance policies provide reimbursement for private sessions.

2. If your child is not meeting the milestones listed above, implement a nutritional approach, such as the Best Dyspraxia Program Ever. In tandem with speech therapy, it may help close the developmental gap.

CHAPTER 17

The Overly Sensitive Child

N OT TOO MANY YEARS AGO, being sensitive was deemed an undesirable trait. When I was growing up, children were frequently corrected (and perhaps even harassed) for crying over an injury or being upset by teasing. "Don't be so sensitive," an adult would snap. If others were present, they would nod in agreement. Rather than being cruel, this was seen as necessary training because life is hard and the strong survive, whereas the sensitive are devoured by the harshness of reality.

Over the last twenty years, our attitudes toward sensitivity have shifted, and it is no longer seen in such black-and-white terms. As a society we recognize that being sensitive to other people's differences and being empathetic is good. But there remains the need for resilience; a child still needs to be able to tolerate the bumps and disappointments of life. Twenty minutes of inconsolable screaming after breaking a leg is accepted as reasonable today, but increasing numbers of children experience the same level of distress when they put on their socks or hear the vacuum cleaner start up.

Some developmental experts claim—and I agree—that these children have sensory processing disorder (SPD), a neurological condition that distorts the way sensory information is read and collated. In SPD, people can be either hyper- or hyporeactive to sensory data in their environment, but the common denominator is that the misreading of information is "off" enough that their reactions and behaviors appear out of sync. Other professionals scoff at the idea of such a disorder. You can almost hear them snap, "Don't be so sensitive." The disorder/not a disorder debate has escalated to the American Psychiatric Association's Diagnostic and Statistical Manual of Mental Disorders (DSM-IV), the main reference used by mental health professionals to classify psychiatric disorders. Advocates expect SPD to appear as an official diagnosis in the next edition. The medical community continues to collect data and debate while the numbers of overly sensitive children skyrocket, and I try to help as many as I can.

SENSITIVE ISAAC

As a baby, Isaac was very sensitive. He cried a lot and was hard to settle. His mother had to tiptoe out of the room when he finally fell asleep, and the slightest noise would start the arduous calming process all over. As long as Isaac was being carried around and his environment was calm and predictable, he was a delight. But the smallest changes caused him big distress, because his capacity for self-soothing was infinitesimal.

"He is just a fussy baby," Isaac's parents were assured by family members with more experience. The pediatrician agreed. There was nothing amiss that she could see. As Isaac blossomed into toddlerhood, his sensitivity did not diminish. He needed constant attention and had zero tolerance for frustration. And there was much to be frustrated about. He could not balance himself and walk until he was seventeen months old. He also had trouble holding a spoon, a sippy cup—even a bottle. He had always been a picky eater, and by age three was restricting his diet to white foods—bread, pasta, cheese, and an occasional chicken nugget.

By the time I met Isaac at five years old, he was still very awkward on the playground and clumsy on structures such as the jungle gym, and even had trouble climbing the ladder of a slide. As with many kids, especially boys, who have trouble with motor skills, this lack of coordination made Isaac feel less than confident socially.

And although he didn't have any language delays (he was actually quite a talker), he did act oddly around other kids, not quite understanding the subtler social cues especially among the boys his age. He had impulse problems and interacted inappropriately with other children. He invaded their personal space and then talked too loudly. To cement his social suicide, he was bossy and always had to win or the meltdowns would commence.

"But he can be so delightful," his mother, Fiona, insisted. And indeed, in my office, Isaac was behaving perfectly. I completely understood the discrepancy between the boy I was looking at and the reports from school. As a mother myself, I also understood Fiona's mixed feelings

---

How Occupational Therapy Became a Hot Field

Twenty-five years ago, pediatric occupational therapists (OTs) concentrated on children with severe disabilities such as spina bifida and cerebral palsy. Now, according to *The New York Times*, OTs have taken their place next to academic tutors, psychologists, and private coaches as part of the large team standing behind academically successful students. Traditionally, they have also stuck to improving non-speech-related skills—fine motor (using the hands), gross motor (whole body), visual perception, and balance/coordination. But now they have branched into skills related to self-regulation: attention, behavior, and emotional flexibility—in other words, the issues surrounding SPD.

Dr. Lynn A. Balzer-Martin is an occupational therapist with a PhD in special education based in Bethesda, Maryland. She consults with pediatricians and is called into preschools to assess children who are having behavior or learning issues to see if the problems are psychological or developmental. Using standardized tests, she determines whether SPD or other causes are behind the troubling behaviors and then recommends the proper treatment.

"SPD is treated using techniques specifically designed to help the child read and organize sensory input effectively and efficiently," she explains to parents. A therapist

about his dual nature. She was aware of both the horrible and wonderful sides to his personality and wanted me not to think too poorly of him even though Isaac needed help. As an adult who did not live in the same house, I thought he was great. He was smart, funny, and engaging when in an ideal situation, i.e., when no other children were present and all of the adult attention was on him. I did not require him to do anything he did not wish to or introduce any stressful activities. Superficial appearances can be deceiving, and I knew he could become unmanageable in a minute should the circumstances shift and make him uncomfortable.

The occupational therapist Isaac's parents had consulted when he was three had diagnosed sensory processing disorder. Since then, he had received regular occupational therapy, which significantly improved his motor planning, although he was still clumsier than other children his age. Unfortunately, his oversensitivity had not responded as well to the therapy. He could handle noises and transitions better, but when he

---

designs specific sensory-based games and activities to indirectly improve the missing or weak skills. For example, a child with a balance problem may play an eye-hand coordination game while swinging on a hammock on her stomach.

"Parents want to know why they should be paying good money to therapists for horsing around with their child," she chuckles. "I explain that sensory integration techniques indirectly improve skills." The terms *sensory integration* and *sensory processing* are used interchangeably by professionals.

Why not just directly teach the specific skill? "Of course, you can improve a specific skill by practicing it over and over," she says, "but then the child only masters that skill in a certain context; they do not necessarily generalize the learning, especially in sensory processing disorder. You would have to practice every separate thing." If a child practices walking in a straight line, she will learn to master walking in a straight line, but she may not be able to walk in that line if there are chairs in the way or a baseball game is going on nearby. Just as soccer practice does not only involve kicking the ball into the goal, first-class sensory processing is not a matter of mastering a handful of individual skills. OTs introduce indirect exercises and play fun games to integrate numerous overlapping processes, with the goal of creating a flexible, well-rounded player at life.

felt the slightest pressure, he pushed back. Pressure could be anything from a child grazing against him on the playground to his mother asking him to put on his coat. Using his advanced verbal skills, he argued about everything with everyone. His teachers were exhausted. Any small request was countered with a ferocious, loud explanation of why he should not have to do what he did not want to do. This control-at-all-costs behavior landed him in the principal's office at least twice a week.

Isaac was bright enough to notice his lack of friends and how he was displeasing the adults around him, but he still could not stop himself. His self-esteem was nonexistent, his academic confidence was crumbling, and the lower he sank, the worse his behavior got. We all rely on our strengths when we do not know how to handle our weaknesses. Isaac had strong verbal skills but weak motor and sensory processing skills. When asked to transition to a new task (a sensory skill) or write (a motor skill), he would simply talk or yell his way out. By the time I was called in, being smart was no longer enough to compensate for Isaac's deteriorating behavior.

SENSORY PROCESSING DEMYSTIFIED

The nervous system is constantly reading and processing thousands of bits of data. How warm or cool are you right now? How much light is in the room? Do you need to use the bathroom? Are you hungry? What is the arm that is not holding this book doing? In order to keep track of the answers to all those questions and thousands more, a complex, well-operating system is required. Not only does the system have to read the data accurately, but the information must be sorted and prioritized so you are immediately aware of only the important stuff. For example, are you hungry right now? No? How about now? Are you hungry now? Of course not. The hunger situation was checked two seconds ago, so there is no need to continuously recheck your appetite or stay focused on eating. When you do get hungry, the nervous system needs to pop the signal to the front of your consciousness so you can order some tandoori chicken. In a well-functioning system, the information is ready and available at the appropriate time.

In kids with SPD, data is misread and/or not collated efficiently, so the information is either wrong, lost among less important information, or not read at all. An example of misreading information is when eight-year-old Patrick head-butts another boy in the class because he is so happy to see him. His potential friend, James, bursts into tears, and Patrick does not understand why James does not want to invite him over to play. What feels to Patrick's sensory system like the right amount of pressure to exert in male-to-male bonding is way over the acceptable limit for most of the other boys of his acquaintance. Patrick is undersensitive to pain and acts according to that wrong information.

For boys, in particular, this is disastrous. According to Dr. Louann Brizendine, author of *The Male Brain*, by the time boys are six, they wrestle, roughhouse, and mock-fight frequently, whereas girls do not. In fact, she observed, boys wrestle, pummel one another, and compete for toys six times more than girls do. This is their social language. Participating in and understanding the physical language allows boys to find their place in the world. For kids with SPD, the physical and sensory signals are constantly misread, so the child is out of sync with what is acceptable pushing and shoving. The rest of the pack will try to provide feedback to correct the behavior, but if the child's sensory system cannot read and adapt to the feedback, he will be pushed out.

> Participating in and understanding the physical language allows boys to find their place in the world. For kids with SPD, the physical and sensory signals are constantly misread, so the child is out of sync with what is acceptable.

Even though Isaac did not have a verbal problem and his motor-planning issues were secondary, I put him on my dyspraxia program (see pages 268–273 in chapter 16), which often helps kids with sensory processing disorder. Recall that fats are structural nutrients, and biochemical support for dyspraxia is fish oil, vitamin E, and choline (preferably as phosphatidylcholine). I also suggested that Isaac take a comprehensive multivitamin/mineral supplement. At a biochemical level SPD is immaturity or underdevelopment of parts of the nervous system, so the three-prong fat support program also works for sensory issues.

What do I mean by nervous system immaturity? When a baby is born, there are plenty of neurons, but they are not interconnected in a complex way. Experiences and learning cause new neuroconnections to be made. This is why babies kept in institutions where they are not touched, carried around, and talked to enough can have brains 25 percent smaller than infants raised in a richer sensory environment. In SPD, there can be experiences, but for reasons not completely understood, the full range of connections in all parts of the brain does not evolve. Although some areas evolve just fine, for kids with SPD, other areas lack the complex neurological circuit-building, resulting in a failure to read and process data efficiently.

THE MANY FACES OF SPD

Because there are so many ways the sensory system can misread signals or fail to process them, SPD can have many manifestations. Here is a sampling of incidents reported by parents of children with SPD.

- Five-year-old Danny's mother reported he had a twenty-minute temper tantrum when she asked him to pick up his hat.

- If there is a fire drill at school, six-year-old Vincent is inconsolable for days. The mother has called the school and keeps him home when they are scheduled.

- Seven-year-old Teisha does not sleep if she knows she has a test at school the next day.

- Nine-year-old Lily yells that everyone hates her when she gets tired and frustrated.

- Four-year-old Megan won't let anyone touch her unless she initiates it.

- Teachers report nine-year-old Leah is fine at school, but her mother says she comes home a mess, picks fights with her sister, and throws things most afternoons.

- Six-year-old Connor cries for thirty minutes if the foods on his plate touch.

SPD AND DIET

What about diet? Isaac was a picky eater. Could switching to a nutrient-rich diet of adzuki beans, sardines, brown rice, and chard with fewer empty-calorie snacks "cure" him? Nutritionists are stereotyped as purveyors of whole food and vegetable pushers, which, as a lot, we are. I talk so much about eating vegetables that I sometimes feel like a faulty iPod replaying the same Usher song. Unfortunately, eating whole food alone is not enough to correct a long-term biochemical mess, especially since kids with SPD rarely cooperate with big dietary changes.

When SPD is involved, the eating problems can be exhausting and overwhelming. Most children with SPD are picky eaters because eating is such a sensory-rich experience. There are smells, colors, flavors, textures, and temperatures, not to mention sights and sounds, involved in eating. Yes, sounds. When you bite into a carrot, it makes a sound. Believe it or not, that bothers some children with SPD. With so many sensations to

---

- Marilyn, eleven, takes one month to adapt to daylight-saving time.

- When something unexpected or stressful happens, ten-year-old Alan will talk repetitively about the event, asking the same questions over and over. "Will there be a fire drill at school tomorrow?" "When is the next fire drill going to be?" "Are you sure it is not tomorrow?" "Maybe you should e-mail my teacher to be sure."

- Three-year-old Noah became very unreasonable and was behaving badly. He did not complain about feeling bad, but whined and cried about everything. A trip to the doctor discovered a ruptured eardrum.

- Seven-year-old Oliver gets hysterical if his mother leaves the room, and follows her all over the house.

- Eight-year-old Bitsy will wear only two pairs of pants. No amount of cajoling can entice her to wear anything else. They are wearing out, and her mother does not know what to do.

- Ben, age seven, still has frequent accidents in his pants. His mother does not know how to stop the behavior, because he can sit in the mess for hours and not seem to notice.

285

experience and interpret, children overload, shut down, and/or try to control the situation.

In mild SPD cases, regular picky eating techniques (see my E.A.T. program on page 52) will work with extra patience and perseverance. For the more severe situations, you first have to find the child under a bundle of disconnected, misfiring neurons. Good luck, sneaky chefs in training. Your child with SPD knows you are thinking about mixing frozen peas in their muffin batter before the freezer door is opened, because he is hypervigilant.

Isaac was one of these hypervigilant kids. For this reason, dietary improvements would take time—time he could not afford to lose in terms of brain development. I started by directly feeding Isaac's nervous system with supplements. Borrowing from *The Jetsons*, an old cartoon about a future where dinner arrives in a pill, we reduced the needed brain nutrients to several teaspoons of liquid. There were the oils from the Best Dyspraxia Program Ever, and I had a pharmacy make up a vitamin and mineral mixture in a flavored base.

Fiona picked the flavor she thought Isaac might tolerate best based on his past inclinations. One convenient aspect of customizing supplements is that the flavor can be changed at will, so if Isaac decided he liked apple better than grape, we could accommodate this sensory preference. The fats were mixed in a sweet, thick base—in this case cinnamon applesauce—and shoveled in like medicine. The vitamins were given straight. We told Isaac what we were doing and did not try to hide the supplements, because he would have noticed. Fiona and I discussed the best incentive program. Isaac would say he would cooperate, but when the time for the new activity finally arrived, he would often balk, so we needed a reason for him to attempt the hard new thing.

Debating and determining how to motivate a particular child is a conversation I have frequently. I need help from parents because I usually do not know the child well enough to choose the best incentive. What worked for Isaac may not work for your sensitive child. He agreed to take the supplements for a week if he could play on his Wii (a video game system) for an extra thirty minutes. (His mother, wisely, restricted his time playing computer games.) He also chose applesauce to put the essential fatty acids in. We added the supplements slowly, so he could adjust to the new routine, and had gotten only the fish oil and multivitamin in by the end of the first week.

Isaac complained a lot at first and decided he wanted to put the EFAs in yogurt instead, but he took everything. He lobbied hard for another thirty-minute session of Wii to continue into week two, and his mom relented because he was adjusting well. You cannot blame kids for pushing back against the new order. Many people need time to adjust to change, and children with SPD especially so. For all of his bravado, Isaac knew he was stuck. But when the nutrients kept showing up, he adjusted. After a transition period of about two weeks, Isaac took everything without comment. Because children with SPD like routine, the hardest part was getting him used to the new requirements. Once on board, he reminded his mother to give him the special mixtures.

SLOW BUT STEADY PROGRESS

Once Isaac started taking the supplements, he started to be slightly more flexible within a few weeks. He was still bossy and difficult, but Fiona noticed that the number of daily incidents was lower. Six weeks after he started the program, his teacher called Isaac's mother to ask if she had changed his diet. Gone was the impulsivity! Gone was the clumsiness! He was also found kissing a girl! This was a kid who had run around unable to interact with his peers.

Isaac also became more flexible about eating. He watched from afar what other kids were eating and now was willing to tentatively taste some new foods. The more he explored, the more interesting foods he discovered. Everyone was surprised to see him shifting away from kid foods and digging into fish and broccoli occasionally. Isaac had lots of school and home support plus years of occupational therapy under his belt, so once the right nutrients were available and the chemistry lined up, he slipped into place. As they say in weight-loss commercials, "This outcome not typical." But in response I would say that I see similar results regularly with a complete program of therapy and nutrients.

BECOMING A FOOD WHISPERER FOR A CHILD WITH SPD

Dog behaviorist and TV star Cesar Millan ("the Dog Whisperer") could have a second career waiting for him. He can take on children with SPD. What he does with dogs works well with these tykes minus the leash. He claims misbehaving dogs are dysregulated and need calm assertion from their owners. Children with SPD cannot regulate their emotions and behaviors, so they depend on the adults around them to do it for them by being calm and assured.

When you think about it, we all do this when possible. If you are having a particularly overwhelming day and find yourself losing control and screaming at the children, how do you calm yourself down? You ask your partner to give you a break, or you look up what parenting experts are saying online, or you call your best friend or mother. All of these techniques involve finding an adult who can help you regulate yourself. You can reason this through and make a plan, but a child with SPD cannot. They cannot comprehend why they are doing what they are doing or how to stop, because the feedback they are getting is confusing and painful and they just want it to stop. Whom are they going to call? Or perhaps scream for or hit? The person they most trust who is available to them: you.

Because sensory input overwhelms them, children with SPD need to control or tune out some of their environment so they can function. They are often described as rigid or control freaks, especially around food. They need to know they can and must eat healthy foods for their own well-being. The mental attitude the parents should exude in their body language is "All is well, you can do this." If the parents lose their tempers and are dysregulated themselves, their behavior adds more fuel to the already overloaded sensory fire. Now everybody is screaming. When parents set an example for how to respond, the child can observe the proper reaction. "I think this food is dangerous and will make me throw up, but Dad seems relaxed," she might note. "Maybe the food is not as bad as I think." Calm assurance is a small but clear step in the right direction. No fighting, no giving up.

Seven-year-old Vivian used to throw a tantrum if her parents dared to ask her to even try a bite of anything. She would get so distressed by the request that she would disrupt the rest of the meal. After years of cajoling, bribing, and sometimes yelling, the family was at a tense stalemate and everyone was upset.

"Stop asking and tell her she needs to take a bite and mean it," I counseled Vivian's mother. Vivian's mom was not calm and assured; she was frazzled and easily thrown off by Vivian's reactions. "You need to be convinced that eating well is as important as going to church or brushing your teeth or whatever else is important enough to you as a parent that you are determined it will get done," I continued.

Feeling sorry for Vivian was not helping her get stronger and overcome this small adversity. Furthermore, Vivian's mother not only felt overly sympathetic but was reacting to her own history of

NUTRITION DETECTIVE
PRINCIPLE #17

Children look to their parents (that's you) to help them regulate.

By age one, most toddlers can fall asleep on their own, which means they have reached the milestone of sleep regulation, and by age four, most preschoolers can recognize and respond appropriately to toileting signals, having reached the developmental milestone of potty training.

Children with SPD cannot read and collate sensory information usefully on their own and need help long past the time when other children have mastered these skills. To cope with these deficits, they attempt to piggyback onto the sensory system of a sympathetic adult. (Alternatively, they disconnect so they appear not to know or care what is happening—your goal is to prevent this from happening.) Recognizing that you are temporarily the external version of your child's internal sensory system will reduce frustration and help you get creative in making a plan to strengthen your child's independent regulation. Typically, developing children also use their parents to help regulate, but not as extensively.

289

food battles with her own mother. She did not like being forced to eat anything as a child and was determined not to do any forcing. Forcing and directing are entirely different, I explained. A parent needs to guide a child about eating decisions or the food companies and kiddie taste buds run unchecked. Talk about what a good diet is and your family values around eating. Do this in small increments, not long lectures. A few sentences here, an observation there. Teaching children about good eating is a long-term project, not a quick lesson. It has to be because their brains cannot integrate huge concepts like what constitutes a good diet. Your children will be hearing about food from myriad sources, so it's better when it comes from you than from your daughter's anorexic best friend or the ads on television.

Directing does not involve forcing children to eat every last bite beyond their natural appetites or forgoing birthday parties. Children's taste preferences should be taken into account when planning meals, but should not rule the entire family. You will have to work to establish good eating habits, with food companies and children's natural taste inclinations toward sweet and salty foods countering you most of the way. As a culture we have allowed children's taste buds to dictate what we buy and how we feed them. The result is cranky, undernourished, and, increasingly, fat children. Time to take back the table.

Armed with new confidence as pack leader, as Cesar Millan would say, Vivian's mom calmly told Vivian she needed to take one bite of a new food every day and that when she was finished, they could read together, as was their after-dinner custom. Vivian started with the same old objections, but when her mother did not back down or get upset, she soon found herself tentatively trying a bite of carrot and then another. Over time Vivian's mother was astonished by how easy it was to shift Vivian's eating once she had calmly decided to take it on.

If you cannot get clear and calm, you may need to examine your own eating behaviors and beliefs before working on your child. Recently, an eating therapist sent me a family who was not progressing well with therapy. "There is no follow-through at home with the exercises," the therapist complained. At the therapy session, the child readily tried the new foods, but the parents couldn't stick to the plan at home.

When I talked directly with the mother, she revealed that she herself did not like any of the recommended practice foods. In fact, the mother was as picky an eater as the child! We had to stop and address these issues first so she could regulate herself around food and then help her child.

Does Your Child Have Sensory Processing Issues?

According to Lindsey Biel, a pediatric occupational therapist and author of *Raising a Sensory Smart Child,* all children have some sensory issues, but parents should be concerned if the behaviors delineated in the questions below are interfering with daily activities and learning. Count up the positive responses to the following:

- ☐ Is your child overly, or under-sensitive to touch, sights, sounds, movement, tastes, or smells?

- ☐ Does your child seem highly distractible? Does he have consistent problems with paying attention and staying focused on a task?

- ☐ Do you consider your youngster to have an unusually high or low activity level?

- ☐ Is frequent tuning out or withdrawing an issue?

- ☐ Does your little one have intense, out-of-proportion reactions to challenging situations and unfamiliar environments?

- ☐ Is difficulty transitioning from activity to activity or situation to situation a big production at your house?

- ☐ Do you sometimes think, "[Child's name] is the most stubborn kid on the planet"? Or do the terms *highly rigid* or *completely inflexible* describe your child too often?

- ☐ Is your child overly clumsy or careless?

- ☐ Does your child show notable discomfort in group situations?

- ☐ Do you think of your child as emotionally immature? Does she act much younger than her age or get along better with younger children?

☐ Is your child overly insecure or awkward? Does she describe herself as "weird" or "stupid"?

☐ Is your child still having tantrums way past the tantrum age? Do her tantrums tend to be longer and more intense than other children's?

☐ Does your child have problems transitioning from an alert, active state to a calm, rested state (for example, difficulty falling asleep or waking, or doing a quiet activity after being very active or vice versa)?

Adapted with permission from *Raising a Sensory Smart Child*, by Lindsey Biel.

If you have answered yes to three or more of these questions, you may be looking at SPD. Biel goes on to explain that children show these signs for a number of reasons, so positive responses alone may not be enough to diagnose SPD. For example, some of these behaviors are appropriate at certain ages, but less so at others. A two-year-old toddler will naturally be impulsive and may pitch a few fits, but a five-year-old who continually acts without thinking may be cause for concern. Exhibiting consistent maladaptive behaviors in everyday situations is the sign that a child needs help.

What to Do

Sensory processing disorder and anxiety are sisters. They are closely related and often travel together. In SPD, anxiety happens when the system overloads and the child is aware enough to know he is overloaded and wants the craziness to stop. Therefore, you may recognize some similar steps between what to do for anxiety and SPD.

1. Have an occupational therapist trained in recognizing sensory issues evaluate your child's individual imbalances and design a program to address his specific issues. Do the suggested exercises regularly. Practice resets a neurological system. Think of it as the neurological fitness program.

2. Children with SPD tend to be picky eaters. Make a commitment to add new healthy foods one at a time, slowly over time. They will drift

toward snack and comfort foods but need regular, balanced meals. Make eating healthfully a priority in your household.

3. Your child with SPD may not be in touch with his hunger and not ask for food even though he needs it. Conversely, he may continue to eat after he is full. Until he develops better internal regulation, you may have to help by setting up regular mealtimes and monitoring portions.

4. Help the nervous system mature by providing good fats in the diet (see chapter 9) and supplemental omega-3 fats. Consider implementing the Best Dyspraxia Program Ever (page 268) if the SPD symptoms are severe or there are motor planning symptoms as well.

THE LIMITS OF NUTRITION

This approach to treating Isaac's SPD worked wonders, but it won't necessarily work for everyone. I used a similar approach with a kid who got kicked out of school because of his unpredictable behavior. Sam was sweet and charming as long as you paid undivided attention to him, but he could also become aggressive for no discernable reason. Unfortunately, no matter how much fish oil, vitamin E, and choline we gave him, Sam's socially inappropriate behavior did not abate. Sam still had violent outbursts and talked about how much he hated himself. His grandmother had brought him to see me, and after several months she reported dejectedly that nothing with Sam had changed; if anything, he seemed to be more agitated and explosive. As the story unfolded, she revealed that Sam's father used to beat his mother in front of him. The father was now out of the picture, but his mother was unable to care for Sam, leaving him with relatives instead. Sam certainly had sensory problems, but nutrition was not going to fix the trauma of witnessing violence against his mother and then being abandoned by both parents. The psychologist who sent him to me was hopeful that a therapeutic nutrition program would help him cope better with a clearly difficult situation, but there were not enough vitamins in the world to fix this legacy of violence.

CHAPTER 18

Frequently Asked Questions

I FIELD QUESTIONS ALL DAY LONG from my clients, doctors, occupational therapists, teachers—you name it: anyone who is the least bit concerned about children's health. The Q and A presented here is a careful culling of the most commonly asked questions and my best responses. As always, trust your own judgment and reach out to a reliable health care practitioner if you have further questions.

I LOVE MY DOCTOR, BUT . . .

1. What should I do if my pediatrician will not go along with a trial elimination diet?

There are two versions of the elimination diet brush-off: "It will never work" and "There is no proof that it works." Both perspectives stem from limited exposure to the wonderful world of nutrition. The best solution is to find an open-minded pediatrician who will partner with you in your diet adventure. The second-best solution is to agree with the doctor that you are not sure the diet will work, but reassert your interest in trying.

Then bring him back into the conversation by asking if there are any medical reasons *not* to do the trial and whether he would agree that a trial is consistent with the medical model of "do no harm." (It should be!)

Usually, at this point, the doctor will admit there is nothing worrisome about the diet except that it might be a waste of your time or money. More nutritionally savvy doctors may express concern over getting enough nutrients, such as calcium if dairy is removed. You can then discuss how to address those issues during the trial period or he can refer you to a nutritionist to help.

Occasionally, a persnickety doctor will insist that the elimination diets or other nutrients you wish to try have been proven not to work. This is a good opportunity to collect data. When this type of situation happens to me when dealing with a doctor, I am tempted to be defensive. Instead, I say, "This is news to me, but it sounds like important information. Could you please give me a copy or refer me to the study so I can read about it?" Do not expect to get anything.

What did happen to me once is that after criticizing me soundly for recommending probiotics, a pediatric GI specialist sent me an entire stack of research. It all supported probiotic use. Attached to it was a note from the specialist. I had irritated him so much, he said, that he decided to do a literature search to show me how unproven my assertions were. Instead, it convinced him that he should use probiotics more proactively with his own patients! He wanted me to know that the research he found was better and more persuasive than what I had to say, so he thought I should have it.

2. How can I find a knowledgeable and sympathetic doctor?

For this question, I talked to my colleague and author of the foreword of this book, Dr. Richard Layton. He gets asked this question a lot because he is a specialist and parents are looking for an understanding pediatrician. His recommended strategy is first to interview the prospective professional. He firmly believes that even if you have to pay for the time, the expense is usually worthwhile. What parents should be looking for is a "comfort zone" with the physician. In other words, he or she should be someone you can talk to easily and trust with the health of your child.

Dr. Layton also suggests avoiding rigid, arrogant physicians who believe nutrition and supplements are unimportant or, worse, "quackery." If your conversation is drifting in this direction, just thank the doctor and leave, he advises. Parents should look for a physician who is willing to be a cocaptain and is empathetic about the child's medical issues. "I think a sympathetic doctor who is willing to admit a lack of knowledge in an area and wants to hear about what is working for you is far better than a know-it-all who is not open to learning," he concludes.

To find a potential sympathetic doctor, talk to friends or other professionals seeing your child. The Internet is a tricky place to locate a good doctor, because many sites with names of professionals are more paid advertising than true patient recommendations. The possible exception is chat rooms where you can ask a lot of questions.

3. I put my son on the same diet and supplement program as my friend; her son got completely better and mine did not do as well. Why is that?

The answer is one word: bio-individuality. Two children can look and act similarly yet have different biological and nutritional needs. The results from the same program can vary from achieving nothing to a miraculous cure in different people. In research, the focus is on finding protocols and solutions that will suit larger target populations. We all like cut-and-dried facts we can depend upon. When you have a sniffle, you want to know for certain which remedy will dry up your nose. We want to know if something works or it doesn't, period. Forget all this "maybe" mumbo jumbo.

Everybody knows that certain drugs and nutrients and medical procedures work for some people and not others, but the idea is uncomfortable nonetheless. Every day somebody asks me if what I am recommending will work. It reminds me of going to a restaurant, and when the waiter recommends something, asking him if it is any good. I catch myself doing this and think, "Why am I even asking such a stupid question? He has no idea what I like—only what most patrons order, what he thinks is tasty, or he is being asked to push."

So I always say, "Yes, it works," and then I add, "but sometimes it doesn't work." Both answers are true, depending on many factors beyond our knowledge and control. The best you can hope to start with is a remedy that works for most of the people most of the time.

VITAMINS AND MINERALS AND SUPPLEMENTS, OH, MY . . .

4. How do I pick a good multivitamin/mineral for my child?

There are several considerations: the quality of the ingredients, the composition of the formula, the fillers and flavors, proper breakdown, and contaminates. Whew! Whole books have been written addressing these various and sundry concerns. Unfortunately, there is no government agency assigned the job of routinely sampling multivitamins/minerals ("multis"), nor are there established standards for what should be in them, so it is all up to the manufacturer who is trying to predict what the consumer will buy. Furthermore, most ingredients are measured as a percentage of a mysterious standard called the Daily Value (DV), and the DVs are general recommendations for what constitutes a healthy diet.

There are two types of daily values. The first is Daily Reference Values (DRVs) for the calorie nutrients such as fat, protein, and carbohydrates, plus additional basic nutrients such as fiber, salt, and potassium. There are values for children over four years of age and these are based on a 2,000-calorie diet. The second type, Reference Daily Intakes (RDIs), are only for vitamins and minerals. The RDIs are based on the National Academy of Sciences' 1998 Recommended Dietary Allowances.

DVs are vague, extremely general ballpark estimates of what might be enough and do not take into account any individual needs. Think of them as a general measure of how much of a nutrient is in a particular product, not as a target number that guarantees optimal health. The RDIs in particular do not always reflect the most recent research. For example, for children, two of the biggest changes in thinking about appropriate daily intake concern vitamin A and vitamin D. Because most children in recent years are low in vitamin D, the old recommended levels are considered way too low. Conversely, vitamin A levels previously considered desirable (about 5,000 IUs) are now thought to be too much for younger children, although some multis still contain high levels.

OTHER FACTORS TO CONSIDER BEFORE PURCHASING A PRODUCT:

1. **Quality of ingredients.** There is no way for an average consumer to evaluate quality of ingredients. You will either have to subscribe to a service that tests supplements, such as www.consumerlab.com, get copies of ingredient verification from the manufacturer (or information about internal quality control), or get the advice of a knowledgeable health care professional. Some products contain a GMP (Good Manufacturing Practices) stamp on the bottle letting the consumer know the company is committed to following certain quality control procedures, or they at least know about them.

2. **Composition of the formula.** The need for nutrients varies greatly between people, depending on their diet, individual metabolic quirks, genetics, medications, age, sex, and medical conditions. In a perfect world, these would all be taken into consideration. To answer the question in general, most multis for kids are weak in minerals. Try to find one that includes zinc, selenium, magnesium, and chromium. These four trace minerals are often lacking in children's diets, and a multi that contains them is usually a better choice and more complete.

   Calcium is almost never present in significant amounts in children's multis. Even in adult multis, you'd need to take three to six pills per day to get a decent amount of calcium, because well-absorbed calcium is bulky and takes up capsule space. If your child does not consume a lot of milk products, expect that he will need a separate calcium supplement.

Ditto for vitamin D. Most children's multis contain 200 to 400 IUs even though most health care professionals now believe 800 to 1,000 IUs are a better goal. To reach the new standards, additional drops or a small capsule of vitamin D3 would have to be added. Vitamin D is called the sunshine vitamin because it can be made when the skin is exposed to sun. Many parents think their children should have enough because they play outside, yet recent studies find that as many as 70 percent of children are low in vitamin D.

Beware of gummy multis. Most of them have an incomplete component of B-vitamins. B-vitamins have a strong flavor and make chewables taste disgusting. To improve the taste, most of the gummies simply do not contain the strongest flavored ones, such as vitamins B1 (thiamine) and B2 (riboflavin), making them poor choices. Be sure the multi you choose contains the full set of B-vitamins (B1, B2, niacinamide, B5, B6, folic acid, and B12).

Finally, take note of fillers/flavors. Fillers tend to be inert but can be a source of trouble when children have allergies or sensitivities. Some multis are made with added wheat, and if a child has a severe gluten sensitivity, he may react to them. Multis can also contain trace amounts of corn, dairy, and other substances. Many of the better companies help by saying "Free of [gluten, dairy, soy, etc.]" clearly on the label.

When possible, avoid artificial colors and flavors. Although the artificial flavors are stronger so they cover the vitamin-y taste better, they can be irritating or cause allergic reactions in young children.

3. **Contaminants.** The most worrisome contaminant occasionally found in vitamins is lead, but luckily this is extremely rare in recent years. Lead is a common mineral and little bits of it are everywhere, so when supplements, food, cosmetics, dishes, or toys are tested, there are often detectable levels. The question becomes: How much is too much? Lead poisoning in children remains a national health crisis, with hundreds of thousands of cases still being identified every year. Cosmetics (such as lipstick), toys, old construction materials in

housing, dishes, and water are the significant causes of lead ingestion. Supplements are not.

5. Why does apple juice work like a laxative in children even though it doesn't have any fiber?

Many parents have noticed that apple juice works like a laxative in children and infants and can even cause diarrhea. Yet if children get diarrhea, parents are told to feed them applesauce! How can apple juice without fiber cause diarrhea yet applesauce with fiber be binding?

Apple juice is very high in fructose. As one researcher put it, "The human fructose absorption capacity has been considerably overrated." When a child starts to exceed her fructose absorption capacity, diarrhea ensues. Children exceed their capacity faster than adults. Applesauce contains the fiber pectin. Pectin can help absorb excess fluid in the colon.

6. What do I do if my child gets worse with a dietary or supplement trial?

The best scenario for an elimination or supplement trial is for everything to get better. The second-best scenario is for symptoms to get worse. By far the worst outcome is no difference. No response means the child is not responsive to that dietary change or supplement, so you are on the wrong track.

Worsening symptoms means you are at least moving along and dealing with something that makes a difference. Stop the trial immediately, of course. Now the challenge is figuring out what the worsening symptom means. Find a medical professional who can help make sense of the situation.

OBSTACLES TO DIETARY CHANGE

7. What if my family/spouse/partner won't go along with my child's dietary changes?

George Burns said, "Happiness is having a large, loving, caring, close-knit family in another city." Short of that, the best strategy is getting them involved in the trial. Tell your family—especially those who help care for your child—that you are making dietary changes for a prescribed period and explain why. Enlist them to help you monitor the experiment and provide feedback about any changes they see or do not see. You may have to provide food or menu ideas for times when the child will be under the family member's care.

If family members absolutely refuse to cooperate or secretly undermine your trial, you need to take a kind but firm stand. Tell them that if it is too much trouble to help, you completely understand, but that you may have to make other arrangements for care or see them less during the test time.

Spouses are trickier, but most go along if you are willing to do most of the work and agree in advance about how long the trial will be. Even if they are not as enthusiastic and do not see the spectacular shifts you do, most join a cooperative effort.

If your spouse absolutely will not go along in any way and the diet is becoming a point of contention, you may wish to consider finding a good psychotherapist. I find that rarely does diet alone deep-six a relationship. Lots of fighting about food usually is part of a bigger pattern of contention. Good therapy teaches partners the skills they need to navigate successfully through disagreements.

8. If my child gets better with dietary elimination and then cheats, will it ruin all of the progress?

Usually not, but in rare instances, yes. In celiac disease, for example, a small cheat will temporarily set back the child, sometimes devastatingly so. More often, there is a short recurrence of symptoms. Some kids can even cheat regularly without ill effect as long as the problem food is mostly out of the diet. Every child is different, so only trial and error will provide an individual answer to this question. It may take several cheats until you see a pattern of ill effects or learn how much of the food can be consumed before eliciting symptoms. There are always confounding factors, because life events happen. Beatrice gets a cold or Edward's birthday party throws him off. Was it the cheese he ate, or too much birthday cake, or staying up too late, or Grandma visiting that caused the regression of symptoms? It takes time to sort all the pieces.

9. What if I cannot see a difference? Should I continue giving my child the supplement or continue with the elimination trial anyway?
With many supplements, you are not supposed to see a difference. Multis, vitamin D, and calcium, for example, are used for health support, and adding them rarely results in immediate, notable improvements in behavior or other noticeable health benefits. Sure, your child may have two fewer cavities than usual at the next dentist visit, but how can calcium and vitamin D use ever be linked to a prevented problem?

Determine which supplements are for all-purpose maintenance and which are being used on a trial basis for a specific reason. Supplements used for a specific reason can cause exciting changes over time, but for the most part, do not expect dramatic improvements in short periods. A 20 or 30 percent improvement is excellent over any period of time, considering the supplements are generally considered safe. Many, such as fish oil, are meant to be used indefinitely.

As for elimination trials, if you do not notice a difference in eight weeks, the food is *probably* not the issue. In some cases, I have had to take out two or three items at the same time before symptoms receded. An irritating food is not the cause of all health problems. Follow your best instincts, and if they do not seem to be solving the problem, get professional help.

10. I took my three-year-old off dairy products and his stuffiness went away and he is sick less often. After a year, I reintroduced some dairy products and he seems fine. Can I just let him have as much as he wants?
You can, but only if you want to go back to the bad old sick days. Not having to be so strict about your son's diet is great news, but doing well with a little dairy is not a license for excessiveness. The prudent approach is to practice moderation. Try a few servings of dairy a week. If that goes well, consider, at most, one serving per day. Watch over several weeks to make sure the stuffiness is not creeping back.

11. *I cannot tolerate milk or soy milk but would like something to put on cereal. Should I use Kelly's Yummy Cow-Free "Milk"?*

I would recommend calcium-fortified almond milk instead! As an adult, the extra protein and fat used to fortify rice or almond milk in my recipe is not necessary. Hopefully, you are getting enough of those nutrients in other parts of your diet. Without dairy products, which are fortified with vitamin D, you may need to add a vitamin D supplement. Finally, cereal with almond milk is a weak, low-protein breakfast. Consider adding some fruit and nuts to your cereal.

RIDICULOUSLY PICKY EATERS

12. *My child will not even allow any new food near his mouth. Even if he eats something he usually likes and it is not quite right, he spits it out. What should I do?*

I talked this question over with my colleague Dianne Lazer, a New Jersey–based speech and language therapist who specializes in eating problems. First and foremost, she suggests having your son checked out by a doctor to make sure he doesn't have any medical conditions that could be responsible for his refusal of healthy food. Also, she strongly recommends finding a nutritionist who can recommend vitamins and supplements so the child gets the nutrients he needs while you work to improve his eating. Changing eating behaviors often takes time.

The next step, she explains, is to slowly introduce the idea of eating the new food by presenting the same food over and over again on a plate that also contains a food he does like. She thinks snack time is best for new food introduction. "Make it a fun time—play board games, read books, or play with toys he loves during these 'therapeutic feedings,'" Dianne says. This is a technique she uses in her clinic.

"What about television?" I asked.

Dianne explains that although television distracts the child, he is not mentally present for learning the new skills.

"For the first few days or weeks, the goal is simply to get him comfortable with smelling or touching the new food. Keep in mind that kids make progress in small steps, so raise the expectations slowly until he is able to keep the food in his mouth and eventually chew and swallow. After he is successful at the 'snack' level, start presenting the same food at mealtimes. Bear in mind that the first new food is the hardest and takes the longest time to integrate into the diet. Your son will know the routine for the second and third foods."

If the child balks, use the "when/then" strategy: "When you eat your bite of food, then you can play outside." (See chapter 4.) He may need some motivation to get over his resistance.

13. How do I know if my child has a problem in her mouth that should be evaluated by an eating specialist?

Some children do not eat because they physically do not have the skills. A parent or therapist can cajole, encourage, or manipulate, but if the basic biting, chewing, and swallowing abilities have not developed, the child simply is not capable. Specific oral motor therapy will be required to help the child build up the necessary skills.

Here are the symptoms of oral motor problems:

- pocketing food in the cheeks
- coughing or gagging while eating
- taking more than thirty minutes to eat a meal
- not increasing food texture variety between one and two years of age
- diagnosis of failure to thrive
- excessive drooling

14. How can I tell if an eating specialist is any good?

I have a list of feeding therapists I recommend to people because this issue comes up so often. All of them have training in a variety of swallowing and feeding techniques and are conscious about introducing healthy foods. They are all certified in their fields (usually either speech or occupational therapy), and most are part of or connected to a multidisciplinary team that also includes other related professionals such as a GI specialist, a nutritionist, or a psychotherapist.

THINKING AHEAD

15. What other conditions or symptoms may benefit from nutritional intervention?

- juvenile rheumatoid arthritis
- obesity
- diabetes
- fatigue
- low muscle tone
- muscle pain/cramps
- mitochondrial disorders
- Down syndrome
- malabsorption syndromes
- Klinefelter's syndrome (when males are born with an extra X chromosome) and other genetic conditions
- precocious puberty
- hormone imbalances
- polycystic ovary syndrome
- cognitive development delays
- memory issues
- a tendency to heal slowly

16. I am not a kid, but I think some of these ideas may apply to me. Is that possible?

Not only is it possible, but it happens all the time. Sometimes I start with a child as the patient and thread the story up through the family, and other times a parent or grandparent is sitting in front of me and we discover that the younger generations share his issues. Nutritional deficiencies or irritations can manifest differently in adults than youngsters: Adults tend to have more autoimmune diseases and fewer ear infections, for example.

The Last Word

"**N**ONE OF THE DIETARY CHANGES are helping," Colleen told me. I had spoken to her for the first time a month earlier, and she wanted me to know she was canceling her follow-up appointment. Her complaint was that the behavior of her son, Forrester, three, was as bad as ever off dairy products *and* (she emphasized) gluten. He was still very hyperactive and hard to manage.

"What about the constipation?" I asked.

That was all gone, she hastily confirmed, trying to get back to her main point.

"His sleep problems?" I persisted.

She admitted they had resolved, but he was still an exhausting child and she did not think nutrition was helping.

I explained to Colleen that nutrition obviously was affecting Forrester's life, just not in the way most important to her yet. She had not tried a sugar-free trial, which I quickly reassured her was completely understandable. Sugar was going to be the hardest item for her to remove in Forrester's case, and she wanted to try eliminating what she deemed the easier foods first. Plus we still needed to look at adding missing nutrients. A person can reasonably make only so many shifts at one time.

At the outset of this book, you may or may not have understood the significant effect that diet can have on the overall health of your child. By this point, as a more informed detective, you may be thinking, "I wonder if fish oil would help Forrester, or perhaps some magnesium?" You will have noticed that some irritants had been eliminated, but you would be curious about how much sugar a three-year-old could be eating if his mother was nervous about removing it. (Way, way too much, as his mother grudgingly admitted.)

If some of these thoughts crossed your mind or, even better, you are thinking about a child you know and love who may benefit from some of these or other nutrition interventions, I have succeeded in my goal for writing this book. It is my hope that as you become more familiar with many of the symptoms, possible causes, and other ways of observing and understanding the health (or illness) of your child, you are growing in confidence as a nutrition detective—even if that confidence only allows you to pick up the phone and get the additional help you need.

In the coming years, I see much of this nutritional information being integrated into standard medical care. Oh, the money and parental agony that will be spared! No longer will we have to wait until children get sick or stop growing or fail to develop cognitively to use such essential information about the power of nutrition to heal and foster optimal health.

But change takes time, and the basic principles discussed here are just an introduction to the possibilities. Colleen and I talked for about fifteen minutes about where Forrester was and what adjustments needed to be made.

"So there is more we can do, right?" Colleen concluded, fishing for some last bit of reassurance.

"More to do?" I replied. "We are just getting started."

References

CHAPTERS 1 AND 2
DETECTIVE THINKING

A. K. Chandler et al., "School Breakfast Improves Verbal Fluency in Undernourished Jamaican Children," *The Journal of Nutrition* 125, no. 4 (1995): 894.

"America's Children: Key National Indicators of Well-being, 2009: Diet Quality."www.ChildStats. gov. A Forum on Child and Family Statistics.

L. S. Freedman et al., "A Population's Mean Healthy Eating Index–2005 Scores are Best Estimated by the Score of the Population Ratio When One 24-Hour Recall Is Available," *Journal of Nutrition* 138 (2008): 1725–1729.

N. J. Goldstein, S. J. Martin, and R. B. Cialdini, *Yes! 50 Scientifically Proven Ways to Be Persuasive* (New York: Free Press, 2008).

P. M. Guenther et al., "Dietary Quality of Americans in 1994–96 and 2001– 02 as Measured by the Healthy Eating Index–2005," *Healthy Insight* 37 (Dec 2007): www.cnpp.usda.gov/ Publications/NutritionInsights/ Insight37.pdf)

A. Hoyland et al., "A Systematic Review of the Effect of Breakfast on the Cognitive Performance of Children and Adolescents," *Nutrition Research Reviews* 22 (2009): 220–243.

S. Moalem and J. Prince, *Survival of the Sickest: A Medical Maverick Discovers Why We Need Disease* (New York: Harper Collins, 2007).

C. A. Powell et al., "Nutrition and Education: A Randomized Trial of the Effects of Breakfast in Rural Primary School Children," *American Journal of Clinical Nutrition* 68 (1998): 873–879.

G. C. Rampersaud et al., "Breakfast Habits, Nutritional Status, Body Weight and Academic Performance in Children and Adolescents," *Journal of the American Dietetic Association* 105, no. 5 (2005): 743–760.

J. Reedy and S. M. Krebs-Smith, "Dietary Sources of Energy, Solid Fats and Added Sugars Among Children and Adolescents in the United States," *Journal of the American Dietetic Association* 110 no. 10 (2010) 1477–1484.

A. P. Smith, "Breakfast and Mental Health," *International Journal of Food Sciences and Nutrition* 49, no. 5 (1998): 397–402.

L. Sanders, *Every Patient Tells a Story: Medical Mysteries and the Art of Diagnosis* (New York: Broadway Books, 2009).

Wesnes et al., "Breakfast Reduces Declines in Attention and Memory Over the Morning in Schoolchildren," *Appetite* 41, no. 3 (2003): 329–331.

CHAPTER 3
PICKY EATING

A. M. Brown and A. P. Matheny Jr., "Feeding Problems and Preschool Intelligence Scores: A Study Using the Co-Twin Method," *American Journal of Clinical Nutrition* 24 (1971): 1207–1209.

The Daily (July 6, 2006) "Canadian Community Health Survey: Overview of Canadians' Eating Habits." www.statcan.gc.ca /daily-quotidien/060706/ dq060706b-eng.htm.

S. M. Krebs-Smith, A. Cooke, A. F. Subar, L. Cleveland, J. Friday, and L. Kahle, "Fruit and Vegetable Intakes of Children and Adolescents in the United States," *Archives of Pediatric and Adolescent Medicine* 150 (1996): 81–86.

G. C. Rampersaud, L. B. Bailey, and G.P.A. Kauwell, "National Survey Beverage Consumption Data for Children and Adolescents Indicate the Need to Encourage a Shift Towards More Nutritive Beverages," *Journal of the American Dietetic Association* 103, no. 1 (Jan 2003): 97–100.

"Parents Shape Whether Their Children Learn to Eat Fruits and Vegetables," *Science Daily* (Aug. 13, 2008). www.sciencedaily.com /releases/2008/08/080811200425 .htm.

CHAPTER 5
REFLUX

L. A. Gupta et al., "Proton Pump Inhibitors and Risk for Recurrent Clostridium Difficile Infection," *Archives of Internal Medicine* 170, no. 13 (2010): 1100.

V. Khoshoo et al., "Are We Overprescribing Antireflux

Medications for Infants with Regurgitation?" *Pediatrics* 120, no. 5 (2007): 946–949 (doi:10.1542/peds.2007-1146).

A. Mahmood et al., "Zinc Carnosine, a Health Food Supplement That Stabilizes Small Bowel Integrity and Stimulates Gut Repair Processes," *Gut* 56 (2007): 168–175.

A. M. Ravelli et al., "Vomiting and Gastric Motility in Infants with Cow's Milk Allergy," *Journal of Pediatric Gastroenterology and Nutrition* 32, no. 1 (2001): 59–64.

F. Savino and E. Castagno, "Overprescription of Antireflux Medications for Infants with Regurgitation," *Pediatrics* 121, no. 5 (2008): 1070 (doi:10.1542/peds.2008-0179).

C. D. Rudolph et al., "Guidelines for Evaluation and Treatment of Gastroesophageal Reflux in Infants and Children: Recommendations of the North American Society for Pediatric Gastroenterology and Nutrition," *Journal of Pediatric Gastroenterology and Nutrition* 32 (Jan. 2001): S1–S31.

A. Fasano, "Surprises from Celiac Disease," *Scientific American* (Aug. 2009): 54–61.

J. D. Godfrey et al., "Morbidity and Morality of Undiagnosed Celiac Disease in Adults Over 50 Years of Age: A Population Based Study," *Gastroenterology* 136, no. 5 (May 2009) A-475.

P. H. Green et al., "Characteristics of Adult Celiac Disease in the USA: Results of a National Survey," *American Journal of Gastroenterology* 96 (2001): 126-31.

M. Kieslich et al., "Brain White-Matter Lesions in Celiac Disease: A Prospective Study of 75 Diet-Treated Patients," *Pediatrics* 108, no. 2 (Aug. 2001): e21.

E. A. Krall and J. T. Dwyer, "Validity of a Food Frequency Questionnaire and a Food Diary in a Short-Term Recall Situation," *Perspectives in Practice* 87, no. 10 (1987): 1374.

A. Rubio-Tapia et al., "Increased Prevalence and Mortality in Undiagnosed Celiac Disease," *Gastroenterology* 137 (2009): 88–93.

CHAPTER 6
GLUTEN INTOLERANCE

E. Barret-Connor, "Nutrition Epidemiology: How Do We Know What They Ate?" *Journal of Clinical Nutrition* 54 (1991): 182S–187S.

Data from the Vital and Health Statistics of the National Center of Health Statistics. Advance Data No. 208, Jan. 17, 1992.

CHAPTER 7
ZINC, GROWTH HORMONE

W. F. Blum et al., "Serum Levels of Insulin-Like Growth Factor 1 (IGF-1) and IGF Binding Protein 3 Reflect Spontaneous Growth Hormone Secretion," *Journal of Clinical Endocrinology & Metabolism* 76 (1993): 1610–1616.

D. R. Clemmons and L. E. Underwood, "Nutritional Regulation of IGF-1 and IGF Binding Proteins," *Annual Review of Nutrition* 11 (1991): 393–412.

T. J. Cole, P. C. Hindmarsh, and D. B. Dunger, "Growth Hormone (GH) Provocation Tests and the Response to GH Treatment in GH Deficiency," *Archives of Disease in Childhood* 89 (2004): 1024–1027 (doi:10.1136/adc.2003.043406).

N. J. Goldstein, S. J. Martin, and R. B. Cialdini, *Yes! 50 Scientifically Proven Ways to Be Persuasive* (New York: Free Press, 2008).

H. Mitchell et al., "Failure of IGF-1 and IGFBP-3 to Diagnose Growth Hormone Insufficiency," *Archives of Disease in Childhood* 80 (1999): 443–447 (doi:10.1136/adc.80.5.443).

A. S. Prasad, "Zinc: the Biology and Therapeutics of an Ion," *Annals of Internal Medicine* 125, no. 2 (July 15, 1996): 142–144.

H. Sandstead, "Zinc Deficiency: A Public Health Problem?" *American Journal of Diseases of Children* 145 (1991): 853–895.

Z. Siklar et al., "Zinc Deficiency: A Contributing Factor of Short Stature in Growth Hormone Deficient Children," *Journal of Tropical Pediatrics* 49, no. 3 (2003): 187–188.

CHAPTER 8
CONSTIPATION

F. Andiran et al., "Cow's Milk Consumption in Constipation and Anal Fissure in Infants and Young Children," *Journal of Paediatrics and Child Health* 39, no. 5 (July 2003): 329–331.

C. C. Cooper, "Probiotics in Pediatrics," *Today's Dietitian* (Jan. 2010): 24–27.

S. Daher et al., "Cow's Milk Protein Intolerance and Chronic Constipation in Children," *Pediatric Allergy and Immunology* 12, no. 6 (Jan. 2002): 339–342.

"Dietary Reference Intakes for Energy, Carbohydrate, Fiber, Fat, Fatty Acids, Cholesterol, Protein, and Amino Acids (Macronutrients)," *Institute of Medicine of the National Academies* (Washington, DC: The National Academies Press, 2005).

D. Goossens et al., "Probiotics in Gastroenterology: Indications and Future Perspectives, *Scandinavian Journal of Gastroenterology* (2003) (Suppl 239).

G. Iacono et al., "Intolerance of Cow's Milk and Chronic Constipation in Children," *New England Journal of Medicine* 339, no. 16 (Oct. 1998): 1100–1104.

B. U. Ling-Nan et al., "Lactobacillus Casei Rhamnosus Lcr35 in Children with Chronic Constipation," *Pediatrics International* 49, no. 4 (2007): 485–490.

E. Miel et al., "Effect of a Probiotic Preparation (VSL#3) on Induction and Maintenance of Remission in Children with Ulcerative Colitis," *American Journal of Gastroenterology* 104 (2009): 437–443.

S. H. Sicherer, "Clinical Aspects of Gastrointestinal Food Allergy in Childhood," *Pediatrics* 111, no. 6 (2003): 1609–1616.

K. S. Sloper et al., "Children with Atopic Eczema. I: Clinical Response to Food Elimination and Subsequent Double-Blind Food Challenge," *Quarterly Journal of Medicine* 80 (1991): 667–693.

A. A. Vass, "Beyond the Grave: Understanding Human Decomposition," *Microbiology Today* (Nov. 2001): 190–192.

CHAPTER 9
ESSENTIAL FATTY ACIDS

N. Auestad, D. T. Scott, and J. S. Janowsky et al., "Visual, Cognitive and Language Assessments at 39 Months: A Follow-Up Study of Children Fed Formulas Containing Long-Chain Fatty Acids to 1 Year of Age," *Pediatrics* 112 (Sep. 2003): e177–e183.

J. R. Chen, S. F. Hsu, C. D. Hsu et al., "Dietary Patterns and Blood Fatty Acid Composition in Children with Attention-Deficit Hyperactivity Disorder in Taiwan," *Journal of Nutritional Biochemistry* 15, no. 8 (2004): 467–472.

W. E. Connor, "Importance of N-3 Fatty Acids in Health and Disease," *American Journal of Clinical Nutrition* 71 (2000) (suppl): 171S–175S.

Data from the National Health and Nutrition Examination Survey (NHANES) reported in *Tufts University Health & Nutrition Letter,* July 2007.

M. G. Enig, *Know Your Fats! The Complete Primer for Undestanding the Nutrition of Fats, Oils and Cholesterol* (Bethesda, MD: Bethesda Press, 2000)

M. Haag, "Essential Fatty Acids and the Brain," *Canadian Journal of Psychiatry* 48, no. 3 (April 2003): 195–203.

I. B. Helland, L. Smith, K. Saarem et al., "Maternal Supplementation with Very-Long-Chain N-3 Fatty Acids During Pregnancy and Lactation Augments Children's IQ at 4 Years of Age," *Pediatrics* 111, no. 1 (Jan. 2003): e39–e44.

J. R. Hibbeln, T. A. Ferguson, and T. L. Blasbalg, "Omega-3 Fatty Acid Deficiencies in Neurodevelopment, Aggression and Autonomic Dysregulation: Opportunities for Intervention," *International Review of Psychiatry* 18, no. 2 (April 2006): 107–118.

H. Nemets, B. Nemets, A. Apter et al., "Omega-3 Treatment of Childhood Depression: A Controlled Double-Blind Pilot Study," *American Journal of Psychiatry* 163 (2006): 1098–1100.

A. J. Richardson, "Omega-3 Fatty Acids in ADHD and Related

Neurodevelopmental Disorders," *International Review of Psychiatry* 18, no. 2 (2006): 155–172.

A. J. Richardson, "Long-Chain Polyunsaturated Fatty Acids in Childhood Developmental and Psychiatric Disorders," *Lipids* 39, no. 12 (2004): 1215–1222.

A. J. Richardson and P. Montgomery, "The Oxford-Durham Study: A Randomized Dietary Supplementation with Fatty Acids in Children with Developmental Coordination Disorder," *Pediatrics* 115, no. 5 (2005): 1360–1366.

A. P. Simopoulos, "Essential Fatty Acids in Health and Chronic Disease," *American Journal of Clinical Nutrition* 70 (1999) (supp): 560S–569S.

M. Singh, "Essential Fatty Acids, DHA and Human Brain," *Indian Journal of Pediatrics* 72, no. 3 (2005): 239–242.

P. Sorgi, E. Hallowell, H. Hutchins, et al., "Effects of an Open-Label Pilot Study with High-Dose EPA/DHA Concentrates on Plasma Phospholipids and Behavior in Children with Attention Deficit Hyperactivity Disorder," *Nutrition Journal* 6 (2007): 16 (doi:10.1186/1475).

V. A. Ziboh, C. C. Miller, and Y. Cho, "Metabolism of Polyunsaturated Fatty Acids by Skin Epidermal Enzymes: Generation of Anti-Inflammatory and Antiproliferative Metabolites," *American Journal of Clinical Nutrition* 71, no. 1 (Jan 2000): 361S–366S.

CHAPTER 10
SLEEP AND MELATONIN

I. M. Anderson et al., "Melatonin for Insomnia in Children with Autism Spectrum Disorders," *Journal of Child Neurology* 23 (2008): 482–485.

G. Coppola et al., "Melatonin in Wake-Sleep Disorders in Children, Adolescents and Young Adults with Mental Retardation with or Without Epilepsy: A Double-Blind, Cross-Over, Placebo-Controlled Trial," *Brain and Development* 26, no. 6 (2004): 373–376.

J. E. Jan, "Use of Melatonin in the Treatment of Paediatric Sleep Disorders," *Journal of Pineal Research* 21, no. 4 (2007): 193–199.

A. Molina-Carballo et al., "Utility of High Doses of Melatonin as Adjunctive Anticonvulsant Therapy in a Child with Severe Myoclonic Epilepsy: Two Years' Experience," *Journal of Pineal Research* 23, no. 2 (2007): 97–105.

Informational overview on melatonin provided by MedlinePlus, a service of the U.S. National Library of Medicine (National Institutes of Health) www.nlm.nih.gov /medlineplus/druginfo/natural /patient-melatonin.html.

N. Peled et al., "Melatonin Effect on Seizures in Children with Severe Neurologic Deficit Disorders," *Epilepsia* 42, no. 9 (2002): 1208–1210.

M. G. Smits, "Melatonin for Chronic Sleep Onset Insomnia in Children:

A Randomized Placebo-Controlled Trial," *Journal of Child Neurology* 16 (2001): 86–92.

M. G. Smits et al., "Melatonin Improves Health Status and Sleep in Children with Idiopathic Chronic Sleep-Onset Insomnia: A Randomized Placebo-Controlled Trial," *Journal of the American Academy of Child and Adolescent Psychiatry* 42, no. 11 (2003): 1286–1293.

M. D. Weiss et al., "Sleep Hygiene and Melatonin Treatment for Children and Adolescents with ADHD and Initial Insomnia," *Journal of the American Academy of Child and Adolescent Psychiatry* 45, no. 5 (2006): 512–519.

CHAPTER 11
SUGAR, ADHD

N. M. Avena et al., "Evidence for Sugar Addiction: Behavioral and Neurochemical Effects of Intermittent, Excessive Sugar Intake," *Neuroscience & Biobehavioral Reviews* 32, no. 1 (2008): 20–39.

J. F. Guthrie and J. F. Morton, "Food Sources of Added Sweeteners in the Diets of Americans," *Journal of the American Dietetic Association* 100 (2000): 43–51.

R. K. Johnson and C. Frary, "Choose Beverages and Foods to Moderate Your Intake of Sugars: The 2000 Dietary Guidelines for Americans–What's All the Fuss About?" *Journal of Nutrition* 131 (2001): 2, 766S–2,771S.

T. Kozielec and B. Starobrat-Hermelin, "Assessment of Magnesium Levels in Children with Attention Deficit Hyperactivity Disorder (ADHD)," *Magnesium Research* 10, no. 2 (June 1997): 143–148.

J. A. Lewis and R. Young, "Deanol and Methylphenidate in Minimal Brain Dysfunction," *Clinical Pharmacol Therapeutics* 17, no. 5 (May 1975): 534–540.

M. Mousain-Bosc et al., "Improvement of Neurobehavioral Disorders in Children Supplemented with Magnesium-Vitamin B6. I. Attention Deficit Hyperactivity Disorders," *Magnesium Research* 19, no. 1 (March 2006): 46–52.

P. N. Pastor et al., "Functional Difficulties Among School-Aged Children: United States, 2001–2007," *National Health Statistics Reports*, no. 19 (Nov. 4, 2009).

O. Re', "2-Dimethylaminoethanol (Deanol): A Brief Review of Its Clinical Efficacy and Postulated Mechanism of Action," *Current Therapeutic Research, Clinical and Experimental* 16, no. 11 (Nov. 1974): 1,238–1,242.

A. J. Richardson and B. K. Puri, "A Randomized Double-Blind, Placebo-Controlled Study of the Effects of Supplementation with Highly Unsaturated Fatty Acids on ADHD–Related Symptoms in Children with Specific Learning Difficulties," *Progress in Neuro-Psychopharmacology and Bio Psychiatry* 26, no. 2 (2002): 233–239.

A. J. Richardson, "Omega-3 Fatty Acids in ADHD and Related Neurodevelopmental Disorders," *International Review of Psychiatry* 18, no. 2 (2006): 155–172.

H. J. Roberts, *Aspartame Disease: An Ignored Epidemic* (West Palm Beach, FL: Sunshine Sentinel Press, 2001).

S. J. Schoenthaler et al., "The Impact of a Low Food Additive and Sucrose Diet on Academic Performance in 803 New York City Public Schools," *International Journal of Biosocial Research* 8, no. 2 (1986): 185–195.

S. J. Schoenthaler, "Los Angeles Probation Department Diet-Behavior Program—An Empirical Analysis of Six Institutional Settings," *International Journal of Biosocial Research* 5, no. 1 (1983): 88–98.

S. J. Schoenthaler, "Diet and Delinquency—A Multi-State Replication," *International Journal of Biosocial Research* 5, no. 2 (1983): 70–78.

N. Sinn and J. Bryan, "Effect of Supplementation with Polyunsaturated Fatty Acids and Micronutrients on Learning and Behavior Problems Associated with Childhood ADHD," *Journal of Developmental and Behavioral Pediatrics* 28, no. 2 (2007): 82–91.

B. Starobrat-Hermelin and T. Kozielec, "The Effects of Magnesium Physiological Supplementation on Hyperactivity in Children with Attention Deficit Hyperactivity Disorder (ADHD). Positive Response to Magnesium Oral Loading Test," *Magnesium Research* 10, no. 2 (June 1997): 149–156.

L. Stevens et al., "EFA Supplementation in Children with Inattention, Hyperactivity and Other Disruptive Behaviors," *Lipids* 38, no. 10 (2003): 1007–1021.

Summary Health Statistics for U.S. Children: National Health Interview Survey, 2006. U.S. Department of Health and Human Services. *Vital and Health Statistics*, series 10, number 234 (Sept. 2007).

R. G. Walton, *Biological Psychiatry* 34, nos. 1–2 (July 1993): 13–17.

CHAPTER 12
GLUTEN/BIPOLAR

K. Bushara, "Neurologic Presentation of Celiac Disease," *Gastroenterology* 128, no. 4 (2005): S92–S97.

G. Gobbi et al., "Coeliac Disease, Epilepsy and Cerebral Calcifications," *The Lancet* 340, no. 8817 (1992): 439–443.

G. Gotti, ed., *Epilepsy and Other Neurological Disorders in Celiac Disease* (New York: John Libbey, 1997).

M. Hadjivassilou et al., "Gluten Sensitivity: From Gut to Brain," *Lancet Neurology* 9 (2010): 318–330.

CHAPTER 13
ANXIETY

Goozner and J. DelViscio, "SSRI Use in Children: An Industry Biased Record" (Feb. 2004): www.cspinet.org/new/pdf/ssri_paper.pdf.

P. Green et al., "Red Cell Membrane Omega-3 Fatty Acids Are Decreased in Nondepressed Patients with Social Anxiety Disorder," *European Neuropsychopharmacology* 16, no. 2 (2005): 107–113.

W. S. Harris et al., "Intakes of Long-Chain Omega-3 Fatty Acid Associated with Reduced Risk for Death from Coronary Heart Disease in Healthy Adults," *Current Atherosclerosis Reports* 10, no. 6 (2008): 503–509.

J. R. Hibbeln, "Fish Consumption and Major Depression," *The Lancet* 351 (1998):1213.

J. L. Jacobson et al., "Prenatal Exposure to Environmental Toxin: A Test of the Multiple Effects Model," *Developmental Psychology* 20, no. 4 (1984): 523–532.

S. Jazayeri et al., "Comparison of Therapeutic Effects of Omega-3 Fatty Acid Eicosapentaenoic Acid and Fluoxetine, Separately and in Combination, in Major Depressive Disorder," *Australian and New Zealand Journal of Psychiatry* 42, no. 3 (2008): 192–198.

K. Kitajka et al., "Effects of Dietary Omega-3 Polyunsaturated Fatty Acids on Brain Gene Expression," *Proceedings of the National Academy of Sciences* 101, no. 30 (2004): 10931–10936.

P. Y. Lin and K. P. Su, "A Meta-Analytic Review of Double-Blind, Placebo-Controlled Trials of Antidepressant Efficacy of Omega-3 Fatty Acids," *Journal of Clinical Psychiatry* 68, no. 7 (July 2007): 1056–1061.

A. C. Logan, "Neurobehavioral Aspects of Omega-3 Fatty Acids: Possible Mechanisms and Therapeutic Value in Major Depression," *Alternative Medicine Review* 8, no. 4 (2003): 410–424.

D. Mozaffarian and E. B. Rimm, "Fish Intake, Contaminants, and Human Health: Evaluating the Risks and the Benefits," *Journal of the American Medical Association* 296, no. 15 (Oct. 18, 2006): 1,885–1,899.

H. Nemets et al., "Omega-3 Treatment of Childhood Depression: A Controlled Double-Blind Pilot Study," *American Journal of Psychiatry* 163 (2006): 1,098–1,100.

Summary of three reports documenting the increase in SSRI prescriptions written for American children: www.neurosoup.com /statisticsonteenssriuse.htm.

"Preliminary Report of the Task Force on SSRIs and Suicidal Behavior in Youth," *American College of Neuropsychopharmacology* (Jan. 21, 2004).

B. M. Ross et al., "Omega-3 Fatty Acids as Treatments for Mental Illness: Which Disorder and Which Fatty Acid?" *Lipids in Health and Disease* 6 (2007): 21.

A. L. Stoll et al., "Omega-3 Fatty Acids and Bipolar Disorder: A Review," *Prostaglandins, Leukotrienes and Essential Fatty Acids* 60, nos. 5–6 (1999): 329–337.

A. L. Stoll, *The Omega-3 Connection* (New York: Simon & Schuster, 2001).

G. Young and J. Conquer, "Omega-3 Fatty Acids and Neuropsychiatric Disorders," *Reproduction Nutrition Development* 45, no. 1 (2005): 1–28.

CHAPTER 14
EAR INFECTIONS

P. Ashwood and J. Van de Water, "A Review of Autism and the Immune Response," *Clinical and Developmental Immunology* 11, no. 2 (2004): 165–174.

J. Fallon, "Could One of the Most Widely Prescribed Antibiotics Amoxicillin/Clavulanate "Augmentin" Be a Risk Factor for Autism?" *Medical Hypotheses* 64 (2005): 312–315.

R. J. Hagerman and A. R. Falkenstein, "An Association Between Recurrent Otitis Media in Infancy and Later Hyperactivity," *Clinical Pediatrics* (May 1987): 253–257.

M. M. Konstantareas and S. Homatidis, "Ear Infections in Autistic and Normal Children," *Journal of Autism and Developmental Disorders* 17, no. 4 (Dec. 1987): 585–594.

K. E. Marconett et al., "Behavior and Developmental Effects of Otitis Media with Effusion Into the Teens," *Archives of Disease in Childhood* 85, no. 2 (2001): 91–95.

T. M. Nsouli, "Role of Food Allergy in Serous Otitis Media," *Annals of Allergy* 73, no. 3 (1994): 215–219.

J. E. Roberts et al., "Otitis Media in Early Childhood and Patterns of Intellectual Development and Later Academic Performance," *Journal of Pediatric Psychology* 19, no. 3 (1994): 347–367.

R. P. Warren et al., "Immune Abnormalities in Patients with Autism," *Journal of Autism and Developmental Disorders* 16, no. 2 (1986): 189–197.

CHAPTER 15
PESTICIDES AND OTHER TOXINS

Alliance for Bio-Integrity, 2040 Pearl Lane #2, Fairfield, Iowa 52556, www.biointegrity.org. This nonprofit, nonpolitical group provides information and advocates for safe and environmentally sustainable technologies. Its website posts scientific position papers and research on GMOs. It also follows lawsuits and regulatory actions regarding GMOs.

D. K. Asami et al., "Comparison of the Total Phenolic and Ascorbic Acid Content of Freeze-Dried and Air-Dried Marionberry, Strawberry and Corn Grown Using Conventional, Organic and Sustainable Agricultural Practices," *Journal of Agricultural and Food Chemistry* 51 (2003): 1,237–1,241.

C. Benbrook et al., "New Evidence Confirms the Nutritional Superiority of Plant-Based Organic Foods" (2008). The Organic Center (www.organic-center.org).

M. F. Bouchard et al., "Attention-Deficit/Hyperactivity Disorder and Urinary Metabolites of Organophosphate Pesticides," *Pediatrics* (doi:10.1542/peds.2009-3058). Published online May 17, 2010.

Environmental Working Group, a nonprofit environmental group based in Washington, DC. For more information, www.ewg.org /node/28365.

R. Harari et al., "Neurobehavioral Deficits and Increased Blood Pressure in School-aged Children Prenatally Exposed to Pesticides," *Environmental Health Perspectives* 118, no. 261 (June 2010).

B. K. Ishida and M. H. Chapman, "A Comparison of the Carotenoid Content and Total Antioxidant Activity in Catsup from Several Commercial Sources in the United States," *Journal of Agricultural and Food Chemistry* 52, no. 261 (2004): 8,017–8,120.

A. R. Marks et al., "Organophosphate Pesticide Exposure and Attention on Young Mexican American Children," *Environmental Health Perspectives* (Aug. 2010).

D. McCann et al., "Food Additives and Hyperactive Behaviour in 3-Year-Old and 8/9-Year-Old Children in the Community: A Randomized, Double-Blinded, Placebo-Controlled Trial," *The Lancet* 370, no. 9598 (2007): 1,560–1,567.

J. S. Newby and C. V. Howard, "Environmental Influences in Cancer Aetiology," *Journal of Nutritional & Environmental Medicine* (2006) 1–59.

R. O'Brien and R. Kranz, *The Unhealthy Truth: How Our Food Is Making Us Sick and What We Can Do About It* (New York: Broadway Books, 2009).

Organic Trade Association website: www.ota.com. Source: "Scientific Frontiers in Developmental Toxicology and Risk Assessment," National Academy of Sciences, National Academy Press, 2000.

P. Rapisarda et al., "Nitrogen Metabolism Components: As a Tool to Discriminate Between Organic and Conventional Citrus Fruits," *Journal of Agricultural and Food Chemistry* 53, no. 7 (2005): 2,664–2,669.

E. M. Roberts, "Maternal Residence Near Agricultural Pesticide Applications and Autism Spectrum Disorders Among Children in the California Central Valley," *Environmental Health Perspective* 115, no. 10 (2007).

D. W. Schab and N. T. Trinh, "Do Artificial Food Colors Promote Hyperactivity in Children with Hyperactive Syndromes? A Meta-Analysis of Double-Blind Placebo-Controlled Trials," *Journal of Developmental and Behavioral Pediatrics* 25, no. 6 (2004): 423–434.

P. W. Stewart et al., "The Relationship Between Prenatal PCB Exposure and Intelligence (IQ) in 9-Year-Old Children," *Environmental Health Perspectives* 116, no. 10 (Oct. 2008).

CHAPTER 16
DYSPRAXIA AND CHOLINE

M. C. Agin, L. Geng, and M. Nicholl, *The Late Talker: What to Do If Your Child Isn't Talking Yet* (New York: St. Martin's Press, 2004).

Z. Cui and M. Houweling, "Phosphatidylcholine and Cell Death," *Biochimica et Biophysica Acta* 1585 (2002): 87–96.

A. Fallbrook et al., "Phosphatidylcholine and Phosphatidylethanolamine Metabolites May Regulate Brain Phospholipid Catabolism Via Inhibition of Lysophospholipase Activity," *Brain Research* 834 (1999): 207.

The Great Courses 2005: "Biology and Human Behavior: The Neurological Origins of Individuality." Taught by Dr. Robert Sapolsky and available through The Teaching Company, Chantilly, VA.

G. C. Lopez and J. R. Berry, "Plasma Choline Levels in Humans After Oral Administration of Highly Purified Phosphatidylcholine (PC) in Capsules," in *Alzheimer's Disease: Advances in Basic Research and Therapies*, ed. R. J. Wurtman et al. Proceedings of the Fourth Meeting of the International Study Group on the Pharmacology of Memory Disorders Associated with Aging, Zurich, Switzerland, Jan. 1987.

J. C. McCann and B. N. Ames, "Is Docosahexaenoic Acid, an N-3 Long-Chain Polyunsaturated Fatty Acid, Required for Development of Normal Brain Function? An Overview of Evidence from Cognitive and Behavioral Tests in Humans and Animals," *American Journal of Clinical Nutrition* 82, no. 2 (2005): 281–295.

National Institutes of Health Dietary Supplement Fact Sheet: Vitamin E. www.ods.od.nih.gov/ FACTSHEETS/VITAMINE.ASP. Updated Dec. 15, 2009.

V. A. Pavlov et al., "The Cholinergic Anti-Inflammatory Pathway: A Missing Link in Neuroimmunomodulation," *Molecular Medicine* 9, nos. 5–8 (2003).

B. J. Stordy, *The LCP Solution: The Remarkable Nutritional Treatment for ADHD, Dyslexia and Dyspraxia* (New York: Ballantine Books, 2000).

R. J. Wurtman and S. H. Zeisel, "Brain Choline: Its Sources and Effects on Synthesis and Release of Acetylcholine," in *Alzheimer's Disease: A Report of Progress*, vol. 19, *Aging*, ed. S. Corkin et al. (New York: Raven Press, 1982).

S. H. Zeisel, "Nutritional Importance of Choline for Brain Development," *Journal of the American College of Nutrition* 23, no. 6 (2004): 621S–626S.

CHAPTER 17
SENSORY PROCESSING DISORDER

L. Biel and N. Peske, *Raising a Sensory Smart Child* (New York: Penguin Books, 2009).

L. Brizendine, *The Male Brain* (New York: Broadway Books, 2010).

P. Tyre, "Watch How You Hold That Crayon," *The New York Times,* Feb. 25, 2010.

CHAPTER 18
FAQ

C. M. F. Kneepkens, "What Happens to Fructose in the Gut?" *Scandinavian Journal of Gastroenterology* 24, no. s171 (1989): 1–8.

Index

321

F

CONTINUE YOUR EDUCATION!

For more information, bonus material, and to follow Kelly's blog, go to www.whatseatingyourchild.com.